Behavior Modification
in
Rehabilitation Medicine

Behavior Modification in Rehabilitation Medicine

By

LAURENCE P. INCE, Ph.D.

Psychology Service, Department of Rehabilitation Medicine
Goldwater Memorial Hospital, New York University Medical Center

CHARLES C THOMAS • PUBLISHER
Springfield • Illinois • U.S.A.

Published and Distributed Throughout the World by

CHARLES C THOMAS • PUBLISHER
Bannerstone House
301-327 East Lawrence Avenue, Springfield, Illinois, U.S.A.

ISBN 0-398-03532-6

Library of Congress Catalog Card Number: 75-40951

With THOMAS BOOKS *careful attention is given to all details of manufacturing and design. It is the Publisher's desire to present books that are satisfactory as to their physical qualities and artistic possibilities and appropriate for their particular use.* THOMAS BOOKS *will be true to those laws of quality that assure a good name and good will.*

Printed in the United States of America
R-1

Library of Congress Cataloging in Publication Data

Ince, Laurence P
Behavior modification in rehabilitation medicine.

Bibliography: p.
Includes index.
1. Physically handicapped--Rehabilitation.
2. Physically handicapped--Psychology. 3. Behavior modification. I. Title. [DNLM: 1. Behavior therapy. 2. Rehabilitation. WM420 136b]
RM930.I45 617 75-40951
ISBN 0-398-03532-6

To Marlene, Valerie and Elizabeth

PREFACE

THE FIELD OF rehabilitation is not a new one, nor is the field of behavior modification. However, a union of these two disciplines is relatively new. Although behavior modification had been successful in many areas of endeavor for several years, it was not until the mid-1960's that its techniques came to be applied consistently to the problems of the physically disabled. Since then, there has been an increasing utilization of behavioral methodologies in rehabilitation institutions. Not only have psychologists carried on this work, but they have trained and encouraged others, such as nurses and therapists, to effectively do so as well. However, much still needs to be done since many rehabilitation professionals are unfamiliar with the principles and methods of behavior modification.

Rehabilitation is a fertile ground for such endeavor for many reasons. Because of the nature of the disabilities of rehabilitation patients, and of the rehabilitation process itself, most patients remain hospitalized for relatively long periods of time. This situation permits greater possible control over their environment than is usually the case in treating human behavior. In addition, there are a great number of variety of behaviors emitted by patients in many diverse settings during rehabilitation hospitalization. Furthermore, the majority of these behaviors, both motor and verbal, are clearly overt and quantitatively specifiable, making for relative ease of observation and measurement. Finally, the goal of rehabilitation and the goal of behavior modification are essentially the same — improved patient functioning. It seems only natural, therefore, that behavior modification methods be extensively employed in rehabilitation settings.

This book is an attempt to unite behavior modification and rehabilitation, by presenting the numerous ways in which behavioral procedures have been employed to benefit rehabilitation patients. It is directed primarily towards the paramedical disciplines such as physical therapy, occupational therapy, speech therapy, psychology and nursing, but there is the hope and the expectation that physicians, social workers, vocational rehabilitation counselors and recreation therapists will see applications to their own fields and benefit from it. It is not intended to be all-inclusive with regard to the literature in the field, but rather to be representative of the work being done. For further study, the interested reader can consult the Appendix, which lists many references not discussed in depth in the text.

For those already knowledgeable in behavior modification, this book may serve to generate new ideas for the application of its techniques to the problems of their patients and motivate them to continue in their work. For those who are unfamiliar with the principles and procedures described herein, perhaps new vistas of treatment will be opened for them.

LAURENCE P. INCE
New York, New York

ACKNOWLEDGMENTS

THERE WERE SEVERAL individuals whose encouragement and support made the writing of this book, while a labor of love, easier and more enjoyable. Not only did many of them express an interest in such a publication and reinforce my thinking on the need, in the field, for a book of this nature, but they freely gave me copies of their work and generously granted permission for the reproduction of materials from their own publications, often on a carte blanche basis.

I wish, therefore, to take this opportunity to thank Victor Benassi, Sidney Bijou, Joseph Brudny, Charles Cleeland, Anthony Fazio, Wilbert Fordyce, Roy Fowler, Bernard Friedlander, Robert Goodkin, David Grove, Richard Herman, Gary Hesse, Anthony Holbrook, R. Don Horner, Irwin Malament, Lee Meyerson, Karl Minke, Mary Mira, J. Grayson Osborne, Thomas Pickering, Alan Roberts, David Roll, David Sachs, Patricia Sand, George Taylor and David Whitten.

I also would like to express my appreciation to the numerous journal editors and publishers who consented to the reproduction of materials acknowledged throughout the text. I am particularly grateful to the American Psychological Association and the American Congress of Rehabilitation Medicine, from whose publications many of the illustrations are drawn.

The reproduction of figures and tables was made possible through the photographic and technical skills of Raoul Hurwitz.

Finally, I want to extend my gratitude to the staff members of the Department of Rehabilitation Medicine of Goldwater Memorial Hospital, who critically listened to or read various portions of the manuscript, improved it through their comments and suggestions, and who, through their progressive attitudes, encourage the use of the procedures described in this volume for the benefit of their patients.

L. P. I.

CONTENTS

SECTION V. BIOFEEDBACK IN REHABILITATION

Behavior Modification
in
Rehabilitation Medicine

SECTION I

ORIENTATION

Chapter One

INTRODUCTION TO BEHAVIOR MODIFICATION

IT IS DIFFICULT to state with certainty precisely when the term *behavior modification* was introduced. Certainly, the basic principles were well known before the term was coined, and the methods were employed prior to their being labelled as *behavior modification* techniques. The early work of Sechenov and Pavlov in Russia, and of Watson, Thorndike and Skinner in the United States, although not directed initially towards therapeutic modification of human behavior, laid the foundations for what we refer to today as behavior modification. As far back as 1924, Jones used conditioning techniques in her extinction of fears in children. In 1938 Mowrer and Mowrer used a behavior modification approach when they treated a problem of enuresis with an operant conditioning procedure, as did Fuller in 1949 to increase arm movements in a profoundly retarded young adult.

While the studies of Jones, Mowrer and Mowrer and Fuller may be viewed as "breakthroughs" in the application of experimental laboratory procedures to human problems, behavior modification as a distinct field of study and treatment received its greatest impetus during the 1950's and early 1960's. There are certain studies which may be considered "classical" which mark the beginnings of the behavior modification "movement," if it can be called such, and which paved the way for the development of the discipline. There will, of course, be disagreements and the reader may feel that the studies cited here are not as "basic" or as important as others with which he is familiar. This is to be expected, since there are no formal criteria for defining a "classical" study. The selection presented herein is based upon the author's opinion, and its arbitrariness is recognized.

In 1955, Greenspoon demonstrated that the techniques of the operant conditioning laboratory, which had repeatedly been found to be effective with animals, could also be successful in modifying the verbal behavior of humans. Flanagan, Goldiamond and Azrin (1958) were able to utilize these methods in controlling stuttering behavior. Ayllon and Michael (1959) not only demonstrated the effectiveness of operant conditioning techniques with psychotics, but also showed that nonpsychologists could be trained to carry out the procedures with the desired results. In 1961, Brady and Lind behaviorally treated a classical neurotic disturbance, hysteria, and Barrett (1962) successfully dealt with a habit disturbance using experimental methodology.

There were also four books whose impact on the developing discipline was significant. Skinner's (1953) *Science and Human Behavior* extended the principles of operant conditioning from the experimental laboratory to a wide variety of complex human behaviors. Wolpe's (1958) *Psychotherapy By Reciprocal Inhibition* set forth, in systematic fashion, a new therapeutic approach based upon psychological learning theory. Bachrach's (1962) *Experimental Foundations of Clinical Psychology* and *Case Studies in Behavior Modification* by Ullmann and Krasner (1965) incorporated both the basic research and the applied aspects of behavior modification. Ullmann and Krasner also defined what is meant by behavior modification and, with regard to viewing human aberrant behavior, clearly differentiated between the traditional medical model approach and the behavioral approach.

Thus, while Jones (1924), Mowrer and Mowrer (1938), and Fuller (1949) provided some of the first examples of behavior modification, it is from the studies and books just cited that the origins of behavior modification can be most clearly traced.

WHAT IS MEANT BY BEHAVIOR MODIFICATION?

The term *behavior modification* actually is self-descriptive. It refers to the modification or alteration of behavior. However, it is not so much the literal definition which sets behavior modification apart as a unique entity, but rather it is its implications which are of greatest significance. These may be listed as follows:

1. The behavior referred to is human behavior.
2. The behavior is usually overt, hence observable and measur-

able.

3. It is the behavior itself which is designated as problemmatical or maladaptive and is not viewed as a symptom of a more fundamental psychic disturbance.
4. The changing of such behavior is beneficial or therapeutic.
5. Modification of the behavior is achieved through the systematic application of certain specific techniques.
6. These techniques are derived from psychological learning theory and/or experimental laboratory evidence.
7. It should be possible to attribute the effected behavior changes directly to the methods employed to bring the changes about.

Thus, while all psychotherapeutic approaches may have the patient's beneficially altered behavior as a goal, not all of the above implications are present, either in their theories or in their methods. It is worthwhile, therefore, to examine some of these implications in detail.

Behavior therapists are concerned with overt and measurable behavior. This does not necessarily imply that covert behavior is not a concern. In fact, as the reader will discover from some of the studies discussed in this book, several techniques are geared to deal with variables which are not immediately seen. Thoughts, feelings, emotions and the like are part and parcel of human existence and cannot be denied or casually dismissed as unimportant. However, ideally, the therapist wishes to be able to observe what he is treating, and he should be able to do so during the course of treatment and upon alleviation of the presenting problems.

Most, if not all covert responses can ultimately be translated into measurable terms. For example, in treating a phobia, the therapist cannot see the feeling of fear which the patient relates to him. However, he can see the patient's behavior when the latter is confronted by the phobic object, can see it become changed during therapy, and finally can note its absence once therapy has been completed. He need never deal with "fear" as a tangible entity. The same may be said for any maladaptive behavior. Measurement plays a crucial role in behavior modification. Unless an accurate measure of a problem behavior is obtained before, during, and after treatment, the therapist can never accurately and fully know the extent of the problem or the effectiveness of his methods in treating it.

Behavior therapists do not view maladaptive behavior as being symptomatic of a "deeper" underlying psychological disturbance. Instead, the problemmatic behavior itself is considered the difficulty to be treated. This psychological approach is in contrast to the dynamic psychotherapies which follow a disease model orientation. In the disease or medical model view, an individual's behavior is considered abnormal because of some presumed but unobserved, underlying cause, much in the same way that a virus produces symptoms in a medically ill patient. Within this framework, the patient's behavior should not be treated directly because it is only a consequence of the underlying psychopathology, and the "real" problem must be dealt with if therapy is to be successful. Thus, much of the patient's actual behavior is ignored while time is spent trying to determine the deep-seated cause which is not apparent, but must be there according to the theory or model. With this viewpoint, should the therapist treat the symptoms directly, therapy will fail because the "root" of the disturbance has not been found and treated, and new symptoms will appear to substitute for those which have been eliminated.

The behaviorist, on the other hand, holds to a psychological model of diagnosis and treatment. This means that he considers the presenting symptoms themselves to be the problem. They are not merely surface manifestations of a more deeply-rooted psychic dysfunction. Hence, they should be treated directly. Without actual evidence of an underlying cause, one should not be assumed. The behaviorist argues that elimination of the undesired behavior does not lead to symptom substitution, and the validity of this argument has been supported by evidence accumulated over many years.

The behavioral model views maladaptive, or aberrant behavior as being learned, and the development and maintenance of such behavior as being no different from that of any other learned behavior. Therefore, since it is learned, it can also be extinguished, or unlearned. A determination must be made of the environmental contingencies which are maintaining the behavior, and these must be modified appropriately so that extinction and new learning can take place.

The techniques of behavior modification were adapted originally from traditional psychological learning theory, primarily the formulations of B. F. Skinner and Clark Hull, or from demonstrated laboratory procedures as developed by Skinner, Hull, Pavlov and their associates. The theories implied certain procedures to test these techniques experimentally, and it was these procedures which were adapted by clinicians for therapeutic application to human problems. (The techniques, such as reinforcement and systematic desensitization, will be discussed at length in ensuing chapters.) As the field of behavior modification grew, new procedures evolved and developed which were not as closely tied to learning theory as were the early approaches, but nonetheless were still founded on basic laboratory principles and methodology.

When therapy is conducted with a patient, the relationship between the therapeutic procedures employed and changes in the patient's behavior should be clearly specifiable. This is important not only for the continuation or abandonment of certain methods for the direct benefit of a given patient, so that the therapist knows which techniques are successful with him and which are not, but also for the possibility of being able to replicate successful procedures with other patients who have similar problems. Not knowing which treatment method is "working" and which is not is to do a disservice both to the patient and to the science.

THE FOUNDATIONS OF BEHAVIOR MODIFICATION

The methodologies of behavior modification can roughly be included within two main categories: those which are based upon operant conditioning and the experimental analysis of behavior, and those based upon Pavlov's classical conditioning and extending from the theories and work of Hull and Wolpe. As the reader continues with this volume, he will become aware that some techniques seem somewhat less closely related than others to either school of thought. As the discipline has grown, new procedures have been developed based upon clinicians' experiences, which may be based only indirectly on Skinner's, Pavlov's, or

Hull's formulations, and which also are successful. Basically, however, the methods of behavior modification do fall within the above-mentioned orientations. The main point to bear in mind is that all methods of behavior modification involve systematic utilization of environmental contingencies to alter the patient's responses to stimuli.

REFERENCES

Ayllon, T. and Michael, J.: The psychiatric nurse as a behavioral engineer. *J Exp Anal Behav, 2*:323, 1959.

Bachrach, A. J.: *Experimental Foundations of Clinical Psychology.* New York, Basic Books, 1962.

Barrett, Beatrice H.: Reduction in rate of multiple tics by free operant conditioning methods. *J Nerv Ment Dis, 135*:187, 1962.

Brady, J. P. and Lind, D. L.: Experimental analysis of hysterical blindness. Operant conditioning techniques. *Arch Gen Psychiatry, 4*:331, 1961.

Flanagan, B., Goldiamond, I., and Azrin, N.: Operant stuttering: The control of stuttering behavior through response-contingent consequences. *J Exp Anal Behav, 1*:173, 1958.

Fuller, P. R.: Operant conditioning of a human vegetative organism. *Am J Psychol, 62*:587, 1949.

Greenspoon, J.: The reinforcing effects of two spoken sounds on the frequency of two responses. *Am J Psychol, 68*:409, 1955.

Jones, Mary C.: The elimination of children's fears. *J Exp Psychol, 7*:382, 1924.

Mowrer, O. H. and Mowrer, W. M.: Enuresis: A method for its study and treatment. *Am J Orthopsychiatry, 8*:436, 1938.

Skinner, B. F.: *Science and Human Behavior.* New York, Macmillan, 1953.

Ullmann, L. P. and Krasner, L. (Eds): *Case Studies in Behavior Modification.* New York, Holt, Rinehart, Winston, 1965.

Wolpe, J.: *Psychotherapy By Reciprocal Inhibition.* Stanford, Stanford Univ. Press, 1958.

Chapter Two

THE METHODS OF BEHAVIOR MODIFICATION

OPERANT CONDITIONING

AN OPERANT IS a behavior, or class of behaviors, which operates on the environment to generate consequences (Skinner, 1953). *Operant conditioning* is a process in which the frequency of occurrence of a bit of behavior is modified by the consequences of the behavior (Reynolds, 1968). In operant conditioning, where the concern is with the relationship between an organism and its environment, the experimental procedure basically involves arranging a reinforcement contingency situation and exposing an organism to it. Rate is the basic datum of operant conditioning, and its techniques are derived from the principles of reinforcement.

Reinforcement

Basic Definitions of Reinforcement

A *positive reinforcer* is any stimulus, contingent upon a response, the presentation of which results in an increase in the frequency of that response occurrence.

Thus, for example, if a physical therapist wishes to reinforce a patient for raising a certain amount of weight to a specified height with pulleys, he can arrange a small switch at the desired height level, which would trigger a bell each time the weight was raised so that it struck the switch, thereby reinforcing that response. If it is desirable for a patient to increase the distance which he ambulates, the therapist can systematically lengthen the distance and reinforce the patient for each advance with a small token, such as a poker chip. A predetermined number of tokens can then be used by the patient to "buy" more time in therapy, or in some other activity which he enjoys.

In both of these examples, correct application of positive reinforcement should produce an increase in the desired behavior.

A *negative reinforcer* is any stimulus, contingent upon a response, the withdrawal of which results in an increase in the frequency of responding.

A hemiplegic patient may discover that positioning his affected arm in a certain way reduces pain in his shoulder. If, in the future, he continues to position his arm that way, the removal of pain is a negative reinforcer which reinforces the response of holding the arm in that position.

It is to be noted that, contrary to the belief of those not familiar with reinforcement techniques, both positive and negative reinforcement increase responding.

Organisms tend to move towards, seek out, and respond in ways to increase the probability of the presentation of reinforcement.

Punishment may be defined as either the withdrawal of a positive reinforcer or the presentation of a negative reinforcer. The effect of punishment is to reduce responding.

When a patient presents a behavior problem such as refusing to perform prescribed exercises, or using foul language in a therapy workshop, he can be punished by the removal of his canteen privileges (withdrawal of a positive reinforcer). If he presents a management problem on his floor or ward by being unusually demanding or hostile to the staff, his bed can be changed to one in a less desirable location (presentation of a negative reinforcer).

Punishment typically produces a fairly immediate suppression of responding, but employing punishment alone is doing only half the job. Once an undesirable behavior has been reduced or eliminated, positive reinforcement of desired behavior should be instituted. Organisms tend to move away from, avoid, and respond in ways which reduce the probability of receiving punishment.

Extinction is the process whereby responses eventually decline in frequency as a consequence of no longer being reinforced.

Many behaviors of patients which are deemed maladaptive or undesirable by the staff actually are being maintained by the staff without their awareness. That is, staff personnel may be reinforcing the very behaviors which they wish to eliminate.

One of the techniques employed to control chronic pain behavior is extinction (Fordyce, 1973). Typically, complaints of pain receive reinforcement in the form of attention from physicians and nurses, medication, and permission to rest from therapeutic exercises. When attention is withdrawn from pain behaviors, when medication is not given contingent upon demand, and when rest is no longer contingent upon complaints — that is, when the pain behaviors are no longer being reinforced — pain behavior is significantly reduced, and often eliminated entirely or extinguished.

Escape and Avoidance Conditioning

In *escape conditioning,* a situation of negative reinforcement, a response terminates an aversive stimulus after the stimulus has begun. The organism can, by making the critical response, escape from or terminate the noxious aspects of the situation.

In *avoidance conditioning,* a response avoids or postpones an aversive stimulus. The organism, by making the correct response, can continually avoid receiving the noxious element of a situation.

In a study conducted by Ince (1969), electric shock was delivered to the nonaffected upper extremity of hemiplegic patients; they could terminate the shock by raising their involved arm a predetermined height. This is an example of escape conditioning. In the avoidance phase of the study, a signal was given prior to the onset of the shock. If the patient raised his arm the required distance during the interval between the signal and the onset of the shock, the timer controlling the shock was reset, thus postponing its onset. The patient, then, avoided the noxious stimulation.

Schedules of Reinforcement

Responses can be reinforced continuously, when each correct response emitted receives reinforcement, or responses can be reinforced intermittently or partially on a reinforcement schedule.

A schedule of reinforcement is the system, or program according to which reinforcement is delivered. The advantages of scheduled reinforcement over continuous reinforcement are mainly two: schedules generate higher rates of responding and behavior maintained on a reinforcement schedule is resistant to extinction.

Simple reinforcement schedules can be classed into two types. Those which require the emission of a certain number of responses for reinforcement to occur are called *ratio schedules.* Those which require that a given time interval elapse before a response is reinforced are termed *interval schedules.*

On a *fixed ratio schedule,* the same total of responses must always be made. Thus, on a fixed ratio schedule of 50, designated as FR 50, only every fiftieth response receives reinforcement. The term *ratio* refers to the ratio of responses to reinforcements. An FR 50 schedule then, delivers one reinforcer for 50 responses.

On a *variable ratio schedule,* the number of responses required for one reinforcement varies in an irregular and usually repetitious manner. The value of a variable ratio schedule is determined by the average number of responses per reinforcement. A VR 50 schedule, therefore, means that every fiftieth response, on the average, is reinforced.

A *fixed interval schedule* requires that a fixed time period elapse before a response is reinforced. A fixed interval schedule of 30 seconds, or FI 30, means that no responses are reinforced during the 30-second period, and that the first correct response emitted after the 30 seconds have elapsed receives reinforcement.

A *variable interval schedule* varies the length of time which must elapse before a response is reinforced. It is summarized as the mean length of time per reinforcement. While on FI 30, the time period remains constant, on VI 30 the first correct response occurring after an average of 30 seconds gets reinforced.

There are many other schedules or reinforcement and combinations of schedules which are employed in operant research (see Ferster and Skinner, 1957) and in applications of operant conditioning. However, the majority of practical applications of operant techniques with humans in nonlaboratory environments make use of one or more of these four basic schedules.

It is important to point out that a reinforcer is defined by its consequences. If the presentation of a stimulus results in increased responding, that stimulus is a positive reinforcer. If the withdrawal of a stimulus increases responding, then that stimulus is a negative reinforcer. If the presentation or the withdrawal of a stimulus has the effect of reducing response rate, those stimuli are punishers. Only when the effects of a stimulus on behavior have been observed can it be classified as either a reinforcer or a punisher.

Shaping

In operant conditioning, a response must occur before reinforcement is delivered. Responses which might not be emitted, or might be emitted only after a considerable length of time, are created by the process known as *shaping*. Shaping is the gradual modification of some property of responses, usually topography, through reinforcement of successive approximations to a final, desired goal (Catania, 1968). Just as a sculptor shapes a piece of clay into its final form of a statue, so the experimenter molds and shapes behavior until it has met the predetermined criteria.

Reinforcement is first given for a response which is similar to or topographically near to the desired response. Then reinforcement is withdrawn and, before the frequency of the behavior decreases, a response which is closer to the desired behavior is reinforced, and so on, each time withdrawing reinforcement from the previous response and making it contingent upon the next closest response to criterion. Finally, only the critical response itself is reinforced.

An example of shaping is provided by Ince (1968) in a study designed to increase the number of positive self-reference statements emitted by subjects. The desired response was a statement which began with the personal pronoun "I," contained no expression of negation, and contained no expression of doubt. At first, all statements which were emitted by the subjects that began with "I" were reinforced, regardless of the content of the remainder of the statement. Next, only statements beginning with "I" and which were free of negation received reinforcement. Finally, only the correct, desired response was reinforced. Thus, step by step, the subjects were conditioned to respond appropriately.

Shaping is necessary not only to generate new behavior, but also to increase rates of responding. If a subject is responding on a continuous (FR 1) schedule of reinforcement and high rates of responding are desired, the subject should be advanced to higher ratios. However, if the schedule shift is made too rapidly, from FR 1 to FR 50, for example, the ratio will be strained and the behavior will extinguish. Therefore, the progression from FR 1 to FR 50 should be made gradually until the final response ratio is achieved. Such a shaping schedule might resemble the following: FR 1, FR 2, FR 4, FR 8, FR 16, FR 26, FR 40, FR 50, or a similar program.

The Baseline

A baseline is a stable, and usually recoverable, level of performance upon which the effects of experimental variables can be assessed. It is the pretreatment behavior. Prior to beginning any experimental or therapeutic manipulation of responding, it is crucial to first measure baseline performance, i.e. how the subject or patient is behaving before the modification technique is introduced. If this is not done, it can never be known conclusively how much of an effect the experimental procedure had on responding.

The baseline period of a study is also occasionally referred to as the *free operant period*. During this phase, the subject(s) responses are observed and recorded. Then the experimental independent variable, such as reinforcement, is introduced. Its effects on performance are noted, and when responding has reached criterion the reinforcement is withdrawn for a period of extinction. If it was, indeed, the reinforcement procedure which modified the behavior, responding should decline in rate to baseline, or near baseline frequency. If other variables were responsible for the altered behavior, responses will be maintained at the higher rate. Thus, baseline measures act as a "check" on the effectiveness of the independent variable.

Determining The Reinforcer

It is difficult, at times, to immediately determine what will be an appropriate reinforcer for any given individual. While animals can be deprived of food or water, and these then can be effectively used to reinforce responding, in working with humans it is obvious that such experimental control conditions usually cannot be created. Therefore, a method is needed to determine which stimuli can effectively be employed as reinforcers without an arduous trial-and-error procedure.

This determination can be made by carefully observing an individual's behavior over a period of time and recording the frequencies with which he engages in the various acts of his daily routine. These behaviors can be arranged in hierarchical order, from those which he engages in least frequently to those which he engages in most frequently. Once this has been done, a high frequency behavior can be used to reinforce one which occurs at a lower rate, but those behaviors which occur at a low frequency cannot be used to reinforce those which have a high rate of occurrence.

Suppose, for example, that there is a patient who spends thirty minutes per day in grooming activities, one hour in occupational therapy, ninety minutes in physical therapy, two hours in speech therapy, and three hours socializing in the hospital canteen. Canteen time can be used to reinforce all other activities, but grooming will reinforce none. Time attending physical therapy can be increased by giving the patient more time in speech therapy, and the patient will spend more time in speech therapy if he is reinforced for it with more free time to socialize in the canteen. While reinforcing grooming with increased occupational therapy time will lead to more grooming behavior, giving the patient more time in occupational therapy will not lead him to spend more time in physical therapy.

Once the reinforcement relationships between behaviors are determined, reinforcement becomes a matter of application. For a more complete description of this reinforcement relationship, the reader is referred to Premack (1959, 1962).

Fading The Stimulus

Fading the stimulus, or simply fading, is a procedure for transferring control of responding from one stimulus, or set of stimuli, to another (Catania, 1968).

If one is teaching shape discrimination to a brain-injured child, geometric shapes can be projected onto a panel of three translucent response keys, each key showing a different shape. Assume that the three shapes are a circle, a square, and a triangle, that each one appears randomly on a different key with each presentation of the figures, and that the child's task is to always press the key on which the triangle is projected. At first, the triangle is colored a bright red, while the circle and the square are simply line drawings. The child will learn to always respond to the shape with the red color. Then, on each successive trial, the color is gradually faded out of the triangle, the red becoming fainter and fainter, until it too is only a line drawing. The child now responds to shape alone. Control of his responding has been transferred from color to form.

Time Out

Time out is a period of nonreinforcement, usually arranged through removal of the opportunity to respond, and thus the preferred behavior receives reinforcement. A disruptive child may be removed from a play situation and placed in another room for a brief time out period where he has no access to reinforcing consequences.

A Final Word On Operant Conditioning

Operant conditioning is a very powerful technique. Its effectiveness has been demonstrated repeatedly over the years in the fields of education and industry as well as in psychology and medicine, with children and adults as well as lower organisms, with the mentally retarded as well as the intellectually gifted, and with the psychologically disturbed as well as those whose behavior would generally be considered as normal.

However, as with any other methodology, the use of operant techniques must be scientific and judicious. No procedure is effective unless it is carried out properly. A sound understanding of the fundamental principles and basic methods is necessary if success is to be achieved. Haphazardly using a technique, no matter how promising that technique is, must inevitably result in failure.

OTHER BEHAVIOR MODIFICATION METHODS

There are a large number and variety of other techniques which are classed under the rubric of behavior modification. Not all of them, however, have been utilized with the physically disabled. This book discusses only two, systematic desensitization and modeling, in its presentation of applied behavioral procedures in rehabilitation. For the interested reader, a list of additional approaches plus references for them is supplied at the end of this section.

Systematic Desensitization

The therapeutic technique known as systematic desensitization is based largely upon the premise that opposing, incompatible feelings cannot exist simultaneously within an individual. One cannot be elated and depressed at the same time, nor simultaneously anxious and relaxed.

In 1938, Jacobson found that deep muscular relaxation inhibits anxiety. Since anxiety is generally considered to be the basis for neurosis, it would therefore seem that if a patient can be taught to relax under conditions which usually arouse anxiety, the anxiety will be inhibited by the relaxation and, eventually, the neurosis will extinguish. As Wolpe (1958) states, "If a response antagonistic to anxiety can be made to occur in the presence of anxiety-evoking stimuli, so that it is accompanied by a complete or partial suppression of the anxiety responses, the bond between those stimuli and the anxiety responses will be weakened." This is, in fact, what occurs.

Systematic desensitization typically involves three main procedures. Initially, a hierarchy of anxiety is constructed by the therapist and the patient. This is a list of situations, or objects, which arouse anxiety in the patient, arranged in order from that which is least anxiety-evoking to that which produces the greatest level of anxiety. The list is compiled and hierarchically-ranked on the basis of the patient's verbal reports, his past history, his responses to inventories such as the *Fear Survey Schedule,* and special investigation into areas of difficulty. The list is constructed so that the progression and spacing of items is appropriate for the particular patient and his problem(s).

An example of such a hierarchy developed to alleviate the fear of flying is as follows:

1. Looking at a photograph of an airplane in a magazine
2. Viewing a three-dimensional slide of an airplane
3. Watching a film of an airplane in flight
4. Driving to an airport
5. Sitting in an airport waiting room
6. Watching airplanes take off and land, from an airport's observation deck
7. Walking towards a grounded airplane
8. Walking up the ramp and entering the airplane
9. Sitting in an airplane while it is on the ground
10. Sitting in an airplane while it is in flight

Next, the patient is trained to relax. This can be accomplished in several ways, including progressive muscular tensing and relaxing, pseudohypnosis or suggestion, hypnosis and drugs, and the training can be conducted by the therapist or by having the patient listen to a taped recording of relaxation instructions. With the exception of drugs, these procedures usually require several sessions before the patient is able to completely relax. He is instructed to practice relaxation between therapy sessions for approximately ten or fifteen minutes per day.

The third phase consists of associating the state of relaxation with imagined or visualized threatening experiences. The therapist requests the patient to envision the items on the hierarchy, beginning with the one which arouses the least anxiety, and proceeding to the item which is most anxiety-evoking. The therapist describes each item or situation in vivid detail, and the patient is instructed to indicate, typically by raising a finger, when he feels anxious or uncomfortable. Each time the patient does so, the presented scene is discontinued, the patient is relaxed, and the item is presented again. This process is repeated until the patient is able to clearly visualize the item without experiencing anxiety. Then the next item on the list is presented by the therapist and the procedure is repeated, and so on until all items on the hierarchy have been desensitized and the patient can clearly visualize the final item without feeling anxious. As each situation on the hierarchy is successively associated with relaxation, a response which is incompatible with anticipated aversive consequences, all of the other items on the hierarchy are affected through generalization.

There is current controversy regarding the necessity for deep muscular relaxation: whether training in muscle relaxation alone effects anxiety; whether hierarchies must be specific to each individual patient, or whether the rate at which a patient can be taken through a given hierarchy can be standardized; and whether a patient should signal anxiety to the therapist verbally or nonverbally (*see* Yates, 1970). The general procedure described above, however, is the one most typically employed in current practice.

Modeling

Modeling, also called vicarious learning, is the technique whereby learning can occur in the absence of the opportunity to perform the responses. The patient observes the behavior of a model, usually the therapist, who is reinforced for correct responding. The behavior exhibited by the model may then be spontaneously reproduced at a later date by the patient under the appropriate conditions, even in the model's absence. Bandura (1965) refers to this as "no-trial learning." Once the patient is under the control of the discriminative stimuli of other people's behavior, these stimuli may be used to alter his future behavior.

In a rehabilitation setting, Goodkin (1966) used modeling in his treatment of an aphasic patient. As the patient observed, Goodkin asked himself the same questions which he had posed in order to elicit responses from the patient. He responded to these questions and both reinforced and punished himself differentially for correct and incorrect responses which he gave by taking the appropriately colored poker chips. Of several techniques which Goodkin employed with this patient, he found modeling to produce the most significant results (see Chapter Five).

ADDITIONAL MAJOR BEHAVIORAL TECHNIQUES

	Selected Readings
Assertive Training	Salter, A.:*Conditioned Reflex Therapy*. New York, Putnam, 1961.
Aversion Therapy	Rachman, S. and Teasdale, J.: *Aversion Therapy and Behaviour Disorders*. London, Routledge, Keegan Paul, 1969.
Aversion-relief Therapy	Thorpe, J. G., Schmidt, E., Brown, P. T. and Castell, D.: Aversion-relief therapy: a new method for general application. *Behav Res Ther, 2*: 71, 1964.
Behavior Rehearsal	Gittelman, M.: Behavior rehearsal as a technique in child treatment. *J Child Psychol Psychiatry, 6*:251, 1965.
Covert Sensitization	Cautela, J. R.: Treatment of compulsive behavior by covert sensitization. *Psychol Rec, 16*:33, 1966.
Covert Therapy	Homme, L. E.: Perspectives in psychology: XXIV. Control of coverants, the operants of the mind. *Psychol Rec, 15*:501, 1965.
Emotive Imagery	Lazarus, A. A. and Abromovitz, A.: The use of "emotive imagery" in the treatment of children's phobias. *J Ment Science, 108*: 191, 1962.
Implosion (Flooding)	Stampfl, T. G. and Levis, D. J.: Essentials of implosive therapy: a learning theory based on psychodynamic behavior therapy. *J Abnorm Psychol, 72*:496, 1967.
Negative Practice	Yates, A. J.; The application of learning theory to the treatment of tics. *J Abnorm Soc Psychol, 56*:175, 1958.

REFERENCES

Bandura, A.: Behavioral modification through modeling procedures. In Krasner, L. and Ullmann, L. P. (Eds): *Research in Behavior Modification.* New York, Holt, Rinehart, Winston, 1965.

Catania, A. C.: *Contemporary Research in Operant Behavior.* Glenview, Scott, Foresman, 1968.

Ferster, C. B. and Skinner, B. F.: *Schedules of Reinforcement.* New York, Appleton-Century-Crofts, 1957.

Fordyce, W. E.: An operant conditioning method for managing chronic pain. *Postgrad Med, 6*:123, 1973.

Goodkin, R.: Case studies in behavioral research in rehabilitation. *Percept Mot Skills, 23*:171, 1966.

Ince, L. P.: Escape and avoidance conditioning of responses in the plegic arm of stroke patients: A preliminary study. *Psychon Science, 16*:49, 1969.

Ince, L. P.: Modification of verbal behavior through variable interval reinforcement in a quasi-therapy situation. *Behav Res Ther, 6*:439, 1968.

Jacobson, E.: *Progressive Relaxation.*Chicago, Univ. Chicago Press, 1938.

Premack, D.: Toward empirical behavior laws. I. Positive reinforcement. *Psychol Rev, 66*:219, 1959.

Premack, D.: Reversibility of the reinforcement relation. *Science, 136*: 255, 1962.

Reynolds, G. S.: *A Primer on Operant Conditioning.* Glenview, Scott, Foresman, 1968.

Skinner, B. F.: *Science and Human Behavior.* New York, Macmillan, 1953.

Wolpe, J.: *Psychotherapy by Reciprocal Inhibition.* Stanford, Stanford Univ. Press, 1958.

Yates, A. J.: *Behavior Therapy.* New York, Wiley, 1970.

SECTION II

APPLICATIONS OF BEHAVIOR MODIFICATION TO MOTOR BEHAVIOR

INTRODUCTION

DEFICIENCIES AND/OR impairments in motor performance are the primary considerations in evaluating a patient's need for rehabilitation. While many patients in a rehabilitation institution may require speech or language therapy, or have psychological problems, or are in need of vocational guidance, these usually are not the crucial reasons for rehabilitative hospitalization, although the patients do receive these services once they are admitted to the hospital. However, if a patient has suffered a cerebrovascular accident and has lost the motoric functions of one side of his body, or has sustained traumatic injury to the spinal cord and is consequently paraplegic or quadriplegic, or has a progressive disease, such as muscular dystrophy or multiple sclerosis, with increasing muscular weakness and/or loss of range of motion, then he is a candidate for rehabilitation.

While a patient is in a rehabilitative setting, the majority of therapeutic efforts are directed at restoring, to as normal a level as possible, lost or impaired motor functioning. In rehabilitation this is the primary responsibility of the physical and occupational therapists. This section is concerned with the utilization of behavioral methodology in these services.

Chapter Three

BEHAVIOR MODIFICATION IN PHYSICAL THERAPY

AMBULATION AND RELATED BEHAVIORS

AMBULATION IS ONE of the more significant activities of rehabilitation. Patients often equate general progress in rehabilitation with the gains they achieve in ambulation, and many patients feel that once they become ambulatory, other impairments they may have will also be alleviated. Although this is, of course, not true, and many patients never become able to ambulate, independent ambulation of a patient is an important goal to work towards whenever possible.

Use of the Tilt Table

It is often the case that prior to receiving training in ambulation, a patient will be required to spend time on a tilt table. This is done to increase circulation and prevent orthostatic hypertension, prevent flexion contractures, facilitate chest expansion, counteract osteoporosis in the lower extremities, provide a change of pressure areas on the body, and prevent loss of the sense of verticality, all of which are important for ambulation.

Frequently, when a patient initially is placed on the tilt table after prolonged bed rest, dizziness and faintness occur, requiring a reduction of the angle of tilt and retarding progress. There are several possible reasons for this, such as a sudden decrease in blood pressure. From a behavioral viewpoint, the patient's complaints of vertigo and syncope may be explained as operants which are being reinforced by the therapist.

This is illustrated by the case of a thirty-three-year-old nurse with incomplete paraplegia (Fordyce, 1968; Fowler, Fordyce and Berni, 1969). As a consequence of skin breakdown in the ischeal areas she had undergone plastic surgery and had been immobilized in bed, postoperatively, for many weeks. When ambulation was finally attempted she became dizzy and faint while trying to walk between parallel bars. Her physician then prescribed a series of sessions on the tilt table preparatory to additional walking. After twenty-eight days, the patient had advanced to a height of 60 degrees but could not tolerate further increases. When raised beyond that level she became faint. At this point, her behavior and that of the therapist were analyzed by the investigators.

Their observations revealed that the typical procedure followed during a therapy session consisted of the physical therapist and an aide placing the patient on the tilt table and, while freely interacting with her, slowly raising the table to an angle which approximated that of the previous day. Then, while keeping the patient under observation, the therapist left her side to perform other duties. After a few minutes, the patient would complain of dizziness and of feeling faint, whereupon the therapist immediately returned to her, lowered the tilt table to the horizontal position, took the patient's blood pressure reading, and reassured her that she was well. The entire procedure then was repeated.

It appeared, therefore, that the therapist's presence and attention were contingent upon the patient's complaints. In addition, the patient's complaining resulted in her being placed in the more comfortable horizontal position. When she was tilted to a more upright position this did not result in attention from the therapist, but, in fact, had the opposite effect of the therapist leaving her, which could be viewed as punishing.

The investigators decided to alter the routine by reversing the contingencies. The therapist was asked to remain with the patient and interact with her throughout the raise toward the upright position. When the patient complained of discomfort, she could be lowered to the horizontal position. The therapist then was to measure her blood pressure routinely and leave her side. When the patient indicated that she was ready to be tilted vertically again, the therapist was to return to her and resume social interaction while elevating the table.

The result of this procedure was that in less than two weeks time the patient ambulated in the parallel bars without any discomfort and no longer required the use of the tilt table. Fifteen days later, she was walking with crutches and was soon discharged from the hospital. The results are illustrated in Figure 3-1.

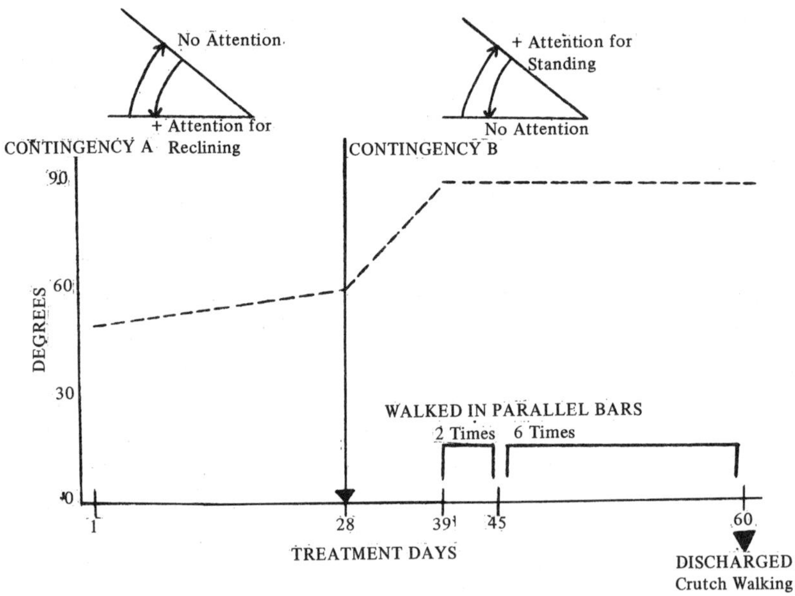

Figure 3-1 Tolerance of elevation on tilt table improved with operant conditioning. From Fordyce, W. E.: The learning model and psychology's role in medical rehabilitation. Paper presented at the Annual Convention of the American Psychological Association, San Francisco, 1968; and Fowler, R. S., Fordyce, W. E. and Berni, Rosemarian: Operant conditioning in chronic illness. *Am J Nurs, June:*1226, 1969.

Reproduced with the permission of the senior authors, the American Psychological Association and the *American Journal of Nursing*. Copyright June, 1969, The American Journal of Nursing Company.

The basic principle adhered to by the investigators was that behavior is largely a function of its consequences. When a response is followed by reinforcing consequences it will be maintained or increased in rate; when it is followed by neutral, or punishing consequences it will decrease in frequency or be eliminated. When the patient's complaints were reinforced by therapist attention and the patient being made more comfortable, they remained at a high rate of occurrence. However, when her complaints were ignored, and positive reinforcement in the form of attention from the therapist was given for desired behavior, the complaints were eliminated and the patient became able to ambulate independently.

Ambulation

Ince (1968) employed verbal reinforcement to improve the ambulation of a fifty-eight-year-old man with Parkinson's disease of several years' duration. The patient ambulated with great difficulty by pushing his wheelchair from behind, using it for support. He exhibited a typical Parkinsonian gait, i.e. stooped shoulders, shuffling, "freezing," slowness, and considerable tremor. In addition, he had little confidence in his ability to ambulate independently and had a chronic fear of falling and hurting himself.

Treatment was conducted during two 1-hour sessions per week in the psychologist's office. The patient was given a series of ambulation tasks to perform, using no assistance of any kind, such as a cane or wheelchair. The tasks were as follows:

1. Rising from a chair.
2. Walking from this chair to a desk on the opposite side of the room
3. Turning about and walking to another desk across the room
4. Walking from that desk to the door of the office
5. Walking from the door to the rear of the office
6. Walking from the rear of the office to the first desk
7. Walking in a circle to the right and returning to starting position
8. Walking in a circle to the left and returning to starting position

All of these tasks involved different distances, ranging from 5 feet to 20 feet, and involved a variety of turns which were very difficult for the patient to make at that time. The eight tasks were performed consecutively.

During the first four sessions, a baseline measure of ambulation time was obtained for each task. The tasks were timed with a stopwatch and a mean walking time was obtained and recorded. On the first experimental day the patient was reinforced verbally for ambulation times which were shorter than the mean times of the baseline period. On each succeeding day he was reinforced for achieving ambulation times which were briefer than those of the preceding day. Reinforcement was delivered immediately upon completion of each task, and consisted of statements by the experimenter such as, "Very good," or "Much better," or "That was better than before," and the like. This form of reinforcement was selected because previous observations of the patient on his ward had revealed him to be highly sensitive to praise and reproof from others. When his performance on a task was the same as, or slower than that of a previous session, reinforcement was withheld and he was told only to go on to the next task.

The patient was seen for a total of four baseline sessions and eleven experimental sessions before he had to be discontinued as a result of developing a severe acute upper respiratory infection.

Task	Operant Period	Experimental Sessions										
	(Sessions 1-4)	5	6	7	8	9	10	11	12	13	14	15
1	60	23	10	24	42	45	11	19	17	4	6	17
2	12	23	8	13	11.5	12.5	11	9	6.5	8	5	5.5
3	57	37	8.5	12	11	34	9.5	19	7	11	9	8
4	19	12	18	13	29	31	18.5	11	12.5	14	9	9
5	63	32	25	16	22	30	20	23	17	20	17	16
6	29	31	19	14	15	13	12	7	11	13	8	6
7	62	42	41	29	45	25	23	26	25	23	30	30
8	126	84	110	57	35	34.5	39	37	60	35	39	33

Table 3-I Rate of ambulation for each task per experimental session. From Ince, L. P.: Behavior modification in a rehabilitation service setting. Paper presented at the Annual Convention of the American Psychological Association, San Francisco, 1968.

The patient's daily performance on each task can be seen in Table 3-I. It can be noted that for the individual ambulation tasks his speed increased markedly from baseline throughout the study.

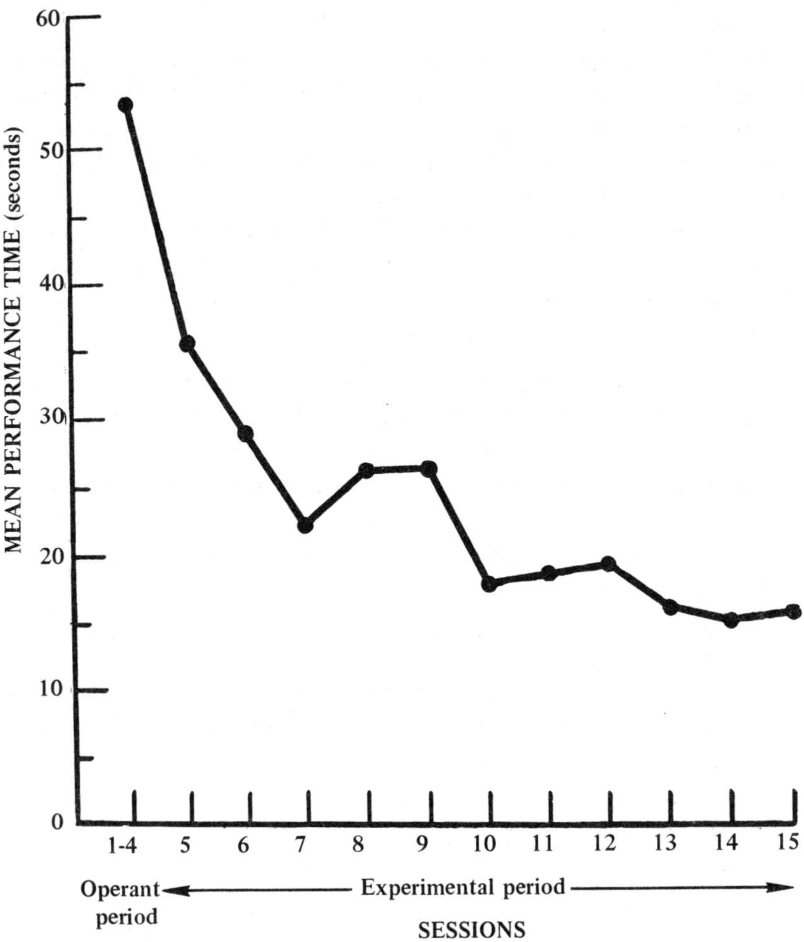

Figure 3-2 Mean performance time for each ambulation task per session. From Ince, L. P.: Behavior modification in a rehabilitation service setting. Paper presented at the Annual Convention of the American Psychological Association, San Francisco, 1968.

Reproduced with the permission of the American Psychological Association.

A comparison of his times on the last experimental day with those of the initial baseline period reveals dramatic improvement on each task. The mean time required by the patient for the eight tasks during the baseline phase was 58.50 seconds, while the mean time for these tasks during the final four experimental sessions was 16.50 seconds.

Figure 3-2 illustrates the patient's mean performance time for all tasks on each experimental day. While there are fluctuations, notable changes can be seen, particularly when comparing his baseline behavior with that of the last few sessions, and his rate of ambulation appears to be stabilizing.

As a consequence of improved ambulation, this man became more self-confident, began to walk about the hospital unaided, and showed a marked improvement of posture and reduction of tremors during ambulation.

A point to be made about this study, and one which arises again in this book, is that it was conducted without the use of any apparatus except a stopwatch, and took place in the psychologist's office. Not all conditioning requires laboratories or sophisticated equipment. While these often are useful, and at times essential, there are many instances when a great deal can be achieved without them.

* * * * *

There are rehabilitation patients who possess the motoric abilities necessary for ambulation, yet who do not do so. In some cases the reasons for this, such as fear of falling, are known, while in others the reasons are less clear. The following studies provide examples of how this type of problem can be dealt with successfully through the utilization of operant procedures.

Horner (1971) worked with a hospitalized five-year-old, moderately retarded boy who had a diagnosis of spina bifida with hydrocephalus and myelomeningocele corrected, and extensive paralysis of both lower extremities. In addition, he had a congenital cerebral defect associated with primary cranial anomaly. Prior to his participation in the operant program he was described as being functionally at the ten month level of motor skills. The child was able to sit, pull to his knees while holding a crib rail, move across the floor in a sitting position and pull himself along while in a prone position.

Following surgery for correction of bilateral hip dislocations he was given high-top shoes and bilateral short-leg braces. Postoperative physical therapy consisted of strengthening exercises for his quadriceps and triceps muscles, and being placed in a sling walker preparatory to ambulation. However, over a six-month period the patient resisted all attempts by the physical therapist to induce him to participate in gait training in parallel bars and with crutches. The therapist's efforts were met with physical resistance and temper trantrums.

Horner's experimental procedure consisted of seven parts: baseline, establishing use of parallel bars, extinction, reinstatement of use of parallel bars, baseline on crutch use, establishing crutch walking, and follow-up. The methodology made extensive use of the technique of shaping, which is described in Chapter Two.

Prior to the baseline period it was determined that root beer was a positive reinforcer, as the child would consistently crawl a distance of 50 feet to receive a tablespoon of root beer in a paper cup. Since he became satiated after 25 spoonfuls, a limit of 25 trials was set for baseline training.

The baseline procedure consisted of providing a verbal request, modeling the requested response once, and repeating the verbal request at intervals of from ten to fifteen seconds. The experimenter sat on a stool between the parallel bars facing the child, who was seated on a stool two feet away. The experimenter instructed the child to "pull up," and placed his hands on the parallel bars, pulling himself to a standing position. No reinforcement was available during the baseline period and responses were scored as to whether or not they were executed within one minute of the demonstration.

Establishing use of the parallel bars consisted of a six-step successive approximation sequence. The steps in the sequence were as follows:

1. Sitting on a stool and gripping the parallel bars with both hands;
2. Pulling to a standing position in the parallel bars and re-

maining in that position long enough to consume a tablespoon of root beer;

3. Taking one step, using the parallel bars;
4. Taking three steps, using the parallel bars;
5. Taking five steps, using the parallel bars;
6. Taking ten steps, using the parallel bars.

Achieving twenty-three successful trials during three consecutive sessions constituted the criterion for progression from one step to the next.

The experimenter sat facing the child, and on each trial he modelled the response once and held the cup of root beer in the position necessary for the reinforcement of a successful response. At ten- to fifteen-second intervals he made the appropriate verbal request. Scoring was performed as it had been during the baseline phase. If the child failed to respond correctly within one minute of the experimenter's demonstration, the cup of root beer was returned to a tray which was placed to the side, away from the parallel bars.

Following the establishment of parallel bar use, an extinction period was introduced where the reinforcer was not present. On each trial the child was requested to perform the behavior established at the end of the training period, i.e. walk ten steps in the parallel bars. This was modelled once by the experimenter, and verbal requests were repeated at intervals of ten to fifteen seconds. After this, the child was given "free" root beer and the procedures used to establish the last step during the training period were repeated.

The treatment procedure for establishing the use of crutches consisted of a ten-step shaping sequence following a baseline period. The successive steps were:

1. The experimenter stood behind the child, and reinforced imitation of the modelled response of placing the crutches on dots marked on the floor 18 inches in front of, and 18 inches from each side of a center line bisecting the starting point;
2. Completion of the first step plus swinging the body to a crutch-supported, erect position, providing total manual assistance. The position had to be maintained for fifteen

seconds in order to receive reinforcement;

3. The same as the second step, with the experimenter providing support only to prime initial movements; (For the first three steps only, the child's hands were secured to the crutches with elastic bandages.)
4. Independently swinging the body to an erect, crutch-supported position;
5. Completion of the fourth step, maintaining balance with the experimenter's hand on the child's back, and placing the crutches in a forward position;
6. Completion of the fifth step plus performing a swing-to gait (see Ince, 1974) and placing the crutches in a forward position;
7. Step six plus one additional cycle of placing the crutches in a forward position, maintaining balance with the experimenter's hand on the back while performing the swing-to, and placing the crutches again in the forward position;
8. Performing four cycles of the above, with gradual fading of the experimenter's support during balancing;
9. Performing eight cycles of the above without any assistance from the experimenter;
10. Performing twelve cycles of the above, using Lofstrand crutches instead of axillary crutches (see Ince, 1974).

From the fifty-fourth session, noise was employed as a reinforcer since it had inadvertently been found to be positively reinforcing for the patient. When he completed a trial successfully he was permitted to use a crutch to strike a dowel holding three weights. This sent the weights crashing to the floor.

The results of the parallel bar training are presented in Figure 3-3. It can be seen that during the baseline period no attempts were made by the child to pull himself up. The first three steps (Steps 0, 1 and 2 on the graph) show rapid acquisition of the desired behaviors. The fourth step (labelled Step 3 on the figure) resulted in 100 percent success on three consecutive days. It took longer to reach criterion in the other steps, partly because the child had difficulty in placing his feet correctly. Extinction resulted in total cessation of the response, but the child immediately responded again in the reacquisition phase.

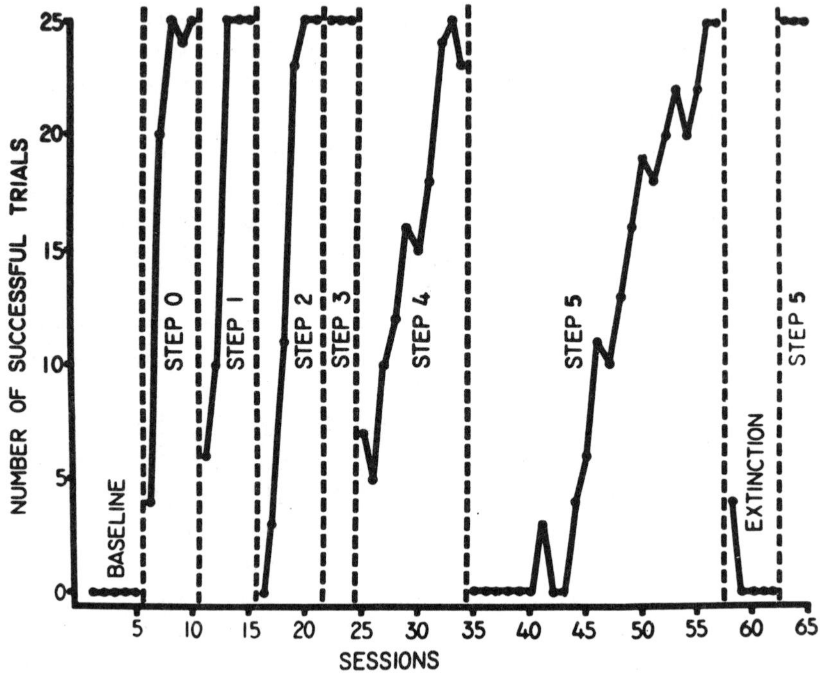

Figure 3-3 Actual number of trials meeting the criterion of the appropriate step within the successive approximation sequence, establishing use of parallel bars over baseline, acquisition, extinction and reacquisition conditions. From Horner, R. D.: Establishing use of crutches by a mentally retarded spina bifida child. *J Appl Behav Anal, 4*:183, 1971.

Reproduced with the permission of the author and the *Journal of Applied Behavior Analysis*. Copyright 1971 by the Society for the Experimental Analysis of Behavior.

Figure 3-4 illustrates the patient's performance in acquiring the use of crutches. As with training in the parallel bars, there was no responding during the baseline sessions. The first two steps in the procedure (labelled Steps 0 and 1 on the figure) required 13 sessions for success to be achieved. The next three steps took 14, 14 and 20 sessions respectively. The next three steps required 13, 11 and 15 sessions, and the final two steps took 12 and 10 sessions to reach criterion.

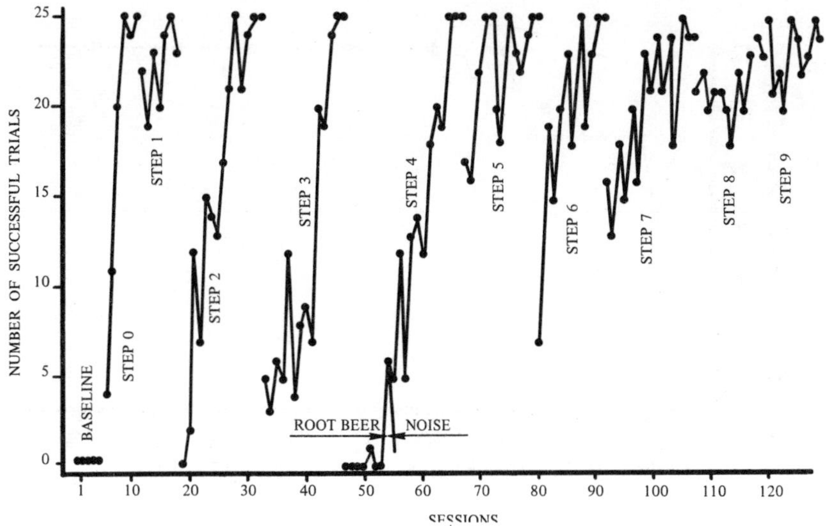

Figure 3-4 Actual number of trials meeting the criterion of the appropriate step within the successive approximation sequence, establishing use of crutches over baseline and acquisition conditions. From Horner, R. D.: Establishing use of crutches by a mentally retarded spina bifida child. *J Appl Behav Anal, 4*:183, 1971.

Reproduced with the permission of the author and the *Journal of Applied Behavior Analysis*. Copyright 1971 by the Society for the Experimental Analysis of Behavior.

The results of a contingency management program designed to maintain crutch usage are shown in Figure 3-5. The figure reveals that the child walked to and from all programs and activities, with only occasional exceptions, within fifteen days posttreatment. Spot checks were made over a fifty-day follow-up period and showed that 100 percent of the patient's twelve opportunities for walking trips per weekday was demonstrated.

The importance of Horner's study lies not only in the obvious gain of enabling a disabled child to achieve ambulation, but also in the researcher's extremely systematized and carefully delineated procedures and in the precision of his measurements. It is precisely for these reasons that the techniques are replicable

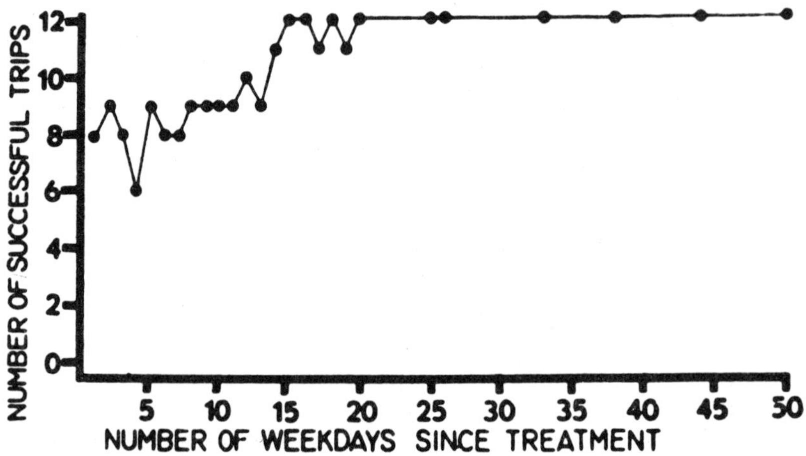

Figure 3-5 Actual number of trips to and from activities successfully completed with the aid of Lofstrand crutches and short leg braces. From Horner, R. D.: Establishing use of crutches by a mentally retarded spina bifida child. *J Appl Behav Anal, 4*:183, 1971.

Reproduced with the permission of the author and the *Journal of Applied Behavior Analysis*. Copyright 1971 by the Society for the Experimental Analysis of Behavior.

and thus applicable to other patients. When progressive steps in a shaping procedure are too large, the response is likely to extinguish. When the description of procedures is too general, or the measurement of responding is too gross, it becomes difficult to understand precisely what was done or achieved, and the value of the study is lost.

* * * * *

Meyerson, Kerr and Michael (1967) employed tokens as reinforcers to overcome the fear of falling during ambulation in a seven-year-old child with mild, spastic cerebral palsy and left hemiplegia. In addition to the primary diagnosis, the patient had nystagmus, ptosis, scoliosis and three-fingered hands without thumbs. Although both his physician and physical therapist believed that he was able to ambulate independently, all attempts to induce him to do so had failed. The child would not walk without holding someone's hand and, in fact, would not even stand unless he was able to hold on to some type of support. He had an extreme fear of falling, but would not do the exercises that would teach him to fall safely without injury.

The psychologists, in making a behavioral analysis of the situation, determined that the adults who were involved actually were reinforcing the child's refusal to ambulate. The considerable attention that he received from those around him for not walking and not doing the falling exercises was enjoyable to him, and hence was maintaining his undesirable behavior.

The goals of the study were set forth as follows: (1) The child should stand and walk independently and learn how to fall safely; (2) The child should ambulate independently to and from the experimental room and should fall, on command, in the proper manner; (3) The child's fear of falling should be overcome and he should experience the freedom of unassisted ambulation so that his behavior could come to be influenced by naturally occurring reinforcers in the environment.

It was believed by the investigators that these behaviors could be established by reinforcement which was more powerful than that which the child was receiving for not walking or not exercising. Since a prior study in which the child had participated had shown him to be highly responsive to token reinforcers which could be exchanged for toys, it was decided to employ such tokens again in the present situation.

As in Horner's (1971) study, a shaping procedure was used. Initially, while the child was engaged in a coloring task, he was given two tokens if he went from his work table to the experimenter's desk and pulled himself up to a standing position. If the experimenter went to the child's table to correct his work, no tokens were dispensed. After only one reinforcement, the child refused to let the experimenter come to him. After twelve reinforcements, he was offered extra tokens for standing at the experimenter's desk without holding onto it. He met this contingency within a single session, and from then on he always stood unassisted.

The second step in the shaping sequence consisted of placing two chairs back-to-back, close enough to each other so that the child could hold onto one chair, turn and grasp the other chair without releasing his grip on the first chair. This, too, was reinforced with tokens. Gradually, the chairs were moved farther apart until he had to release the first chair and take one or more steps to get to the second chair. By the end of the first session, he had walked three unassisted steps from one chair to the other.

Five days later, the child walked into the experimental room for his next session, unassisted. His verbal behavior revealed that the ambulation itself had become reinforcing for him and he now was ambulating independently about the institution.

The next phase of the program focused on having the child learn to fall safely and properly upon command. His physical therapist felt that his incoordination, resulting from the spastic paralysis, would probably result in occasional falls, and that it would be beneficial for him to learn to fall correctly without injury or discomfort.

The experimenters treated the falling behavior by subdividing it into successive approximations to the final goal. The steps involved were:

1. Placing the child's hands and knees on a mat and having him roll to one side;
2. Placing him on his knees with his body upright on the mat, and having him first fall forward onto his hands and then roll to one side;
3. Standing the child beside the mat and having him first fall to his knees, then onto his hands, and then roll to one side.

The child was informed of the procedure and was shown the steps to be performed. Tokens then were made contingent upon his performing the desired behaviors on command.

As Table 3-II shows, success was achieved in only four 20-minute sessions. Once rolling behavior had become established, the other steps were conquered rapidly. The authors additionally report that the child engaged in the behaviors willingly, and almost eagerly, with none of the emotionality that had been associated with previous attempts to teach him to fall correctly in physical therapy classes.

		Responses	
Sessions (20 minutes)	Rolling to side	Falling from knees to hands and rolling	Falling from upright to knees, hands and rolling
1	8	3	---
2	2	2	7
3	3	---	4
4	---	5	6

Table 3-II Frequency of the component parts of the falling sequence during four sessions of training. From Meyerson, L., Kerr, Nancy and Michael, J.: Behavior modification in rehabilitation. In Bijou, S. W. and Baer, D. M.: *Child Development: Readings in Experimental Analysis*. New York, Appleton-Century-Crofts, 1967.

This study illustrates the importance of carefully specifying, at the outset, the treatment program, the goals and the methods of achieving them. While it may become necessary because of unforeseen events to alter a program once it is in progress, no research, basic or applied, nor therapy can be entered into without a previously well-delineated plan. Carrying out procedures as they "come to mind" is doomed to failure.

It should additionally be noted that Meyerson and his associates made a behavioral analysis of the problem before they decided upon their methodology. Behaviors do not occur without reason. The environmental contingencies which are maintaining a behavior or set of behaviors should be determined whenever possible if a meaningful treatment plan is to be developed. Often, the very behaviors which are deemed undesirable are actually being maintained by environmental reinforcers. This was seen in the studies of Fordyce (1968) and Fowler, Fordyce and Berni (1969), which have been previously discussed. A behavioral analysis will reveal this, and thereby enable the investigator to appropriately modify the contingencies so that success may be achieved.

* * * * *

Refusal to ambulate because of a fear of falling was treated in a different manner by Di Scipio and Feldman (1971).

A fifty-two-year-old woman had exhibited progressively deteriorating symptoms of Parkinson's disease over a seven-year period prior to being treated by the investigators. Following eighteen months of supportive treatment in the hospital, including chemotherapy and group psychotherapy for anxiety neurosis, she became severely bradykinetic and confined herself to a wheelchair, expressing a morbid fear of falling.

Systematic desensitization was selected as the method of choice for overcoming this fear. A hierarchy was constructed, consisting of five situations in which the patient might fall, either in the presence of aides or alone. Ten sessions of relaxation training conducted over a two-week period were required for the patient to achieve a satisfactory state of relaxation. Relaxation was not complete because of her disease-related tremors.

The hierarchy items were progressively worked through until the final item elicited no anxiety from the patient. A total of seven desensitization sessions were conducted during a period of three weeks.

Following this treatment the patient's physical therapist reported considerable progress, evidenced by reduced bradykinesis and an ability to ambulate with a walker. The patient's verbal reports and self-report anxiety scales, which were administered following each desensitization session, indicated a general reduction of fears related to falling and participation in physical therapy.

The authors state that a brain lesion generally is considered as a contraindication for this type of behavior therapy, but the results in this case appear to imply otherwise.

An interesting aspect of this study is that despite the fact that complete, deep muscle relaxation was never achieved because of the rigidity and tremor produced by the patient's disease, the desensitization procedure was effective. It has been pointed out (Rachman, 1968) that reciprocal inhibition of anxiety may be accomplished if the patient achieves a state of calm. Apparently, that is what occurred in this case, and the results are promising for similar therapy with other patients whose disease or disability precludes total muscular relaxation.

Wheelchair Propulsion

Although ambulation is always the desired goal to be reached with the physically disabled patient whenever feasible, there are many patients who, because of the severity of their handicaps, will never be able to walk despite the best efforts of a physical therapy service. These individuals must come to accept the fact that they will remain wheelchair-bound, and must learn to function maximally at this level of mobility. There are many activities to be learned in wheelchair use (see Ince, 1974), one of the most important being locomotion, that is, propelling the wheelchair from place to place independently. Some patients will not do this because it is an arduous, fatiguing, and often frustrating task, and thus they become dependent upon others for their mobility. Goodkin (1966) successfully dealt with a case of this nature.

A sixty-one-year-old woman with Parkinson's disease had the strength and range of motion necessary to propel her own wheelchair, yet refused to perform the activity. She stated that she felt there was no use in trying because even small children could push their wheelchairs along faster than she could. Observation of this patient revealed that she actually put forth very little effort in her attempts to propel her wheelchair and spent most of her time complaining to her physical therapist that she could not do the task.

Prior to working with this patient, Goodkin laid strips of red tape down on the floor of a large room at five-foot intervals for a distance of twenty feet.

The patient then was seen for twenty-minute sessions each day. Each trial consisted of having her propel her wheelchair forward for a distance of five feet. On the first day, a baseline measure was obtained of the amount of time it took her to do this. A one-minute rest period followed every trial.

Treatment began on the second day. Each trial was timed and recorded, and the times of the trials were averaged at the end of every session. The patient was reinforced for faster times by telling her that she was doing well, telling her the number of seconds it took her to traverse five feet, and informed her of how many seconds she had cut off her previous time. When she performed more slowly she was told nothing. Each day, she received her initial reinforcement after the first response, which was faster than the mean time of the previous day. At the end of the session the patient was informed of her average time for the session, and this was compared with that of the previous sessions. In addition to being a reinforcing, this had the effect of getting her to focus more on her own performance and less on comparing herself with others.

Trials (5 ft.)	Day 1	Day 2	Day 3
1	32	25	17
2	20	19	15
3	25	17	22
4	29	23	20
5	24	15	20
6	19	17	16
7		20	15
8		15	17
9			16
10			21
11			17
Total	149	151	196
M	24.8	18.9	17.8

Table 3-III Response time (in seconds) to propel a wheelchair a distance of five feet. From Goodkin, R.: Case studies in behavioral research in rehabilitation. *Percept Mot Skills, 23*:171, 1966.

Reproduced with the permission of the author and *Perceptual and Motor Skills.*

The patient was seen for just three days, a total of eleven trials, before she was discharged from the hospital. The results are presented in Table 3-III. Each day the patient spontaneously requested that she be given additional trials, and each day she propelled her wheelchair faster.

* * * * *

Goodkin's study was a pioneering effort, and like that of Ince (1968) required almost no apparatus. A somewhat more sophisticated research design was employed by Grove (1970) in dealing with a similar problem.

Two female patients, aged ten and sixteen years, and one male patient, aged eleven years, all with varying degrees of spastic quadriparesis and athetosis, did not propel their wheelchairs despite having the physical capabilities for doing so.

Grove mounted a small, reset, ratchet-drive, mechanical counter on the patients' wheelchairs. A counter-activating arm was attached to a wheel of each chair, so that each revolution of the wheel activated the counter once. Additionally, a lever was attached to a pushing handle of each wheelchair which, when depressed, prevented the counter from recording. This was done so that the counter would record only the self-movement behavior of the patients and would not count wheel revolutions when they were being pushed by someone else. Staff were requested to depress the lever whenever they pushed the patients about.

There were three main phases to the experiment. In Phase I, a baseline of the patients' self-movement of their wheelchairs was obtained. At the beginning of each physical therapy session, the counters of their wheelchairs were set at zero, and the wheel of the chair was turned so that a revolution of at least 180 degrees was required to activate the counter. At the end of each session the counters were read, the data was recorded, and the counters were reset to zero. (Counts were converted later to distance travelled.) Two 30-minute sessions per day were conducted for the duration of the study. The baseline period was continued until the patients' behavior had stabilized.

In Phase II, at the end of each session and before resetting the counter, the experimenter said to each subject, "Look at your counter. You have *X* amount of counts on it." The purpose of this was to determine if this alone would significantly effect the patients' baseline rates. A multiple baseline was used throughout the study, whereby experimental manipulations were applied to one patient at a time while the others acted as controls. When a behavioral change was demonstrated with one patient, the same treatment was given to another patient while the previous patient was maintained at the newly achieved rate.

Phase III introduced the reinforcement. Reinforcement was in the form of verbal praise, e.g. "Good," "Good for you," and was contingent upon activation of the counter. Every response received reinforcement. A response was defined as a one-quarter revolution of the wheel. This was increased to a greater revolution requirement each time responding stabilized at a particular level, until fading of the reinforcement could be carried out. Fading was accomplished by changing the reinforcement schedule from one of continuous reinforcement (FR 1) to variable interval schedules of increasing interval lengths.

When the data indicated that the verbal reinforcement could not maintain the patients' behavior, a fourth phase was added on the same schedules, in which primary reinforcers such as food were employed.

The data for the three patients involved in this study are shown in Figure 3-6. The patients are indicated by P1, P2 and P3. Each data point represents a thirty-minute therapy session. Responses are plotted in one-quarter revolutions of the wheel.

The first patient averaged 3.0 responses during the baseline condition, and the addition of the verbal statements in Phase II increased responses to only 3.8. In Phase III she increased her responses to a high of 24.0 per session and stabilized at that level. The requirement for reinforcement was raised from one-quarter revolution of the wheel to one-half revolution and responses increased to 38.0 per session. Then they declined to 4.0 and food was substituted for verbal praise as the reinforcer. This resulted in an increase of 47.8 responses over the next nine sessions. When the criterion for reinforcement was raised to a three-quarter turn of the wheel, responding decreased slightly to a mean of 42.0 responses per session over thirteen sessions, but because behavior had stabilized, the reinforcement requirement was raised to one full revolution of the wheel. Over the next thirteen sessions the patient's rate of responding averaged 76.0 per session, with a high total of 120.0 responses during a single session.

At this point reinforcement was withdrawn to demonstrate the

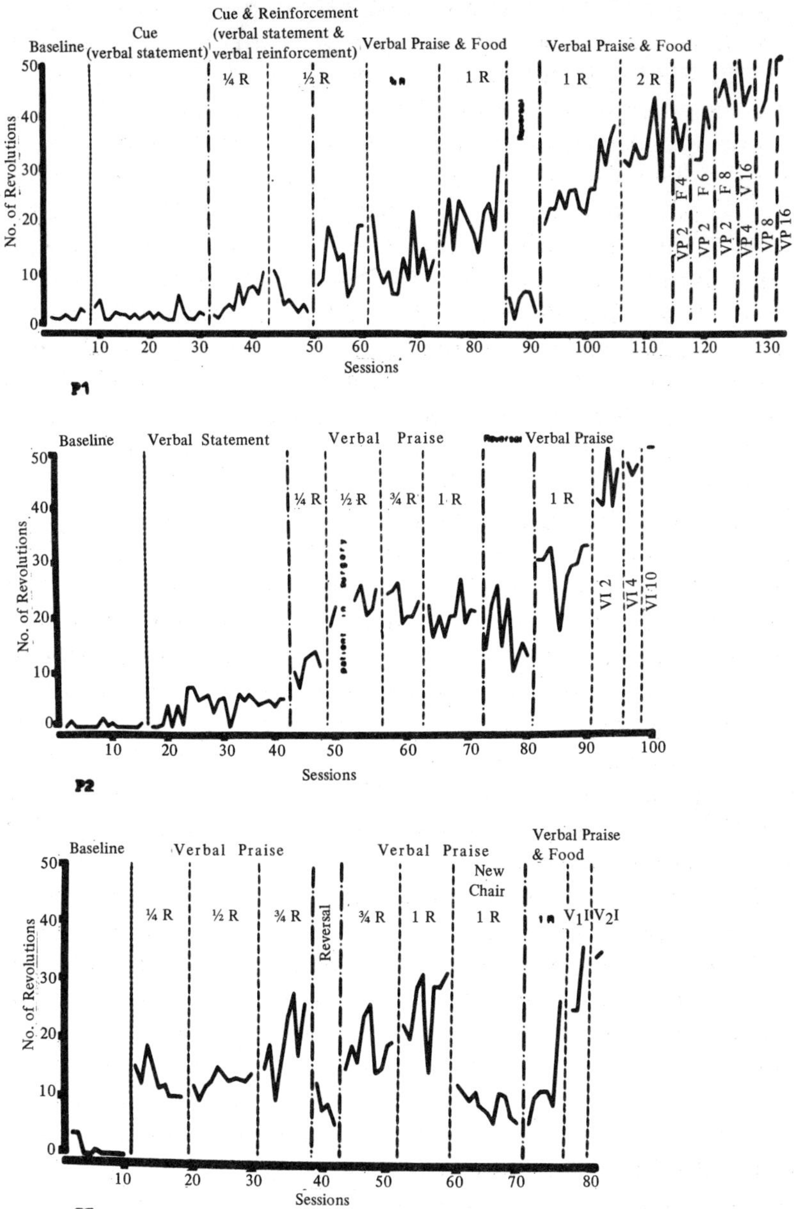

Figure 3-6 Wheelchair self-mobility. From Grove, D. N.: Application of behavioral technology to physical therapy. Paper presented at the Annual Convention of the American Psychological Association, Miami Beach, 1970.

Reproduced with the permission of the author and the American Psychological Association.

causal effect of the procedure. Six extinction sessions were conducted and responses decreased to a mean of 12.7 per thirty-minute session. Reinforcement then was reintroduced, resulting in a mean response rate of 98.0 for fifteen sessions.

The response-reinforcement criterion was raised to two revolutions of the wheel and the patient averaged 131.6 responses over the next nine sessions. Then, verbal praise was used as a reinforcer for every two revolutions of the wheel, but food was delivered on schedules of FR4, FR6 and FR8. The patient's mean responses under these schedules were 108.0, 139.0 and 169.3 respectively.

The second patient, labelled P2 in the figure, produced a mean of 0.8 responses during the baseline phase. In Phase II this was increased to 15.0 responses over twenty-six sessions. Introduction of the verbal reinforcer in Phase III resulted in a mean of 45.8 responses over six sessions for the quarter-turn requirement, and 74.0 responses for the half-turn requirement. After the patient had been lost to the study for five weeks due to needed surgery, she returned and reestablished her responding at a mean of 92.0 per session. A change to the three-quarter turn requirement for reinforcement produced an average of 90.0 responses per session over seven sessions. This was followed by the one complete revolution contingency, extinction, and return to one full revolution. Responses during these steps averaged 83.4, 63.1 and 107.6, respectively. Reinforcement then was scheduled as VI2′, VI4′ or VI10′, and the mean number of responses per session increased to 190.6 at the VI10′ condition.

Baseline data for the third patient, P3, showed a mean of 2.9 responses per session in the baseline phase. Phase II was not included for this subject mainly because of its minimal effects with the other two subjects. In Phase III, the one-quarter revolution criterion produced a mean of 47.4 responses per session. The one-half revolution requirement increased responding to an average of 51.0 responses per session; increasing the contingency requirement to a three-quarter turn produced further increases in responding to a mean of 80.6 for eight sessions. Extinction resulted in a decrease in response level to 36.0 per session over four sessions, and a steady decline to 24.0. Reintroduction of the reinforcement resulted in an increase to 79.0 responses per thirty-minute session.

This study demonstrates not only the capability of an operant conditioning procedure to instate an important behavior, but additionally, to increase and maintain that behavior over long periods of time. While the apparatus and recording methods employed by Grove were effective, he points out that they were very time consuming and that a telemetry system, used concurrently with a solid-state decoding, recording and automated reinforcing system would be superior in terms of saving time and repairs.

Grove's is an example of a well designed conditioning procedure carefully applied to a therapeutic endeavor. It involves several basic operant conditioning techniques, including baseline measurement, shaping by successive approximations, schedules of reinforcement and extinction, and clearly demonstrates the cause-and-effect relationship between procedures and responding.

Posture

Good posture is important not only for disabled persons, but also for the prevention of disabilities in the nonhandicapped. Our bodies are continually subjected to the force of gravity, and while this force is utilized in equilibrium and movement, it simultaneously places stress on the body structures responsible for maintaining the upright position. Thus, postural defects are common and many individuals suffer from some type of distress or disability because of strain and injury to antigravity structures, some persons becoming disabled to the extent that rehabilitative efforts become necessary. In addition, in planning for an effective program of ambulation, a patient's posture must be evaluated, since good posture is important for good gait.

To date, there is a paucity of studies on the modification of postural problems in rehabilitation. It is worthwhile, however, to mention two studies which dealt with the correction of posture in nondisabled persons, since the techniques employed by the researchers appear to be directly applicable to rehabilitation patients.

Azrin, Rubin, O'Brien, Ayllon and Roll (1968) worked with

twenty-five adults, both male and female, in an effort to reduce slouching. Slouching was defined behaviorally as a sustained rounding of the shoulders or upper back while in a standing position.

The experimenters mounted a miniature snap-action switch, modified to operate when pulled, on the back of each subject at the level of the first, second or third thoracic vertebra. The switch was connected to an elastic cord and attached to the back so that rounding of the back resulted in closure of the switch contacts. Fifteen of the subjects had the attachment mounted with adhesive tape, and ten subjects used a harness-type attachment. A three-second closure of the switch defined the response.

A 500 cycles per second (cps) tone at an intensity of 55 decibels (db) was the stimulus consequence for slouching. The tone was generated by a transistor circuit which included a hearing aid speaker. The onset of the tone constituted a punisher for slouching, and termination of the tone served as escape reinforcement for the cessation of slouching. A warning stimulus of a "click" from the posture switch preceeded the onset of the tone by three seconds if the switch remained closed.

The posture switch arrangement was connected by a thin lead wire that passed loosely under the shirt to the programming device, which was suspended from a cloth necklace. The male subjects wore the apparatus under their shirts, and the female subjects typically wore it in their brassieres. The apparatus weighted 60 g, and measured 2 X 4 X 6 cm. It contained the mercury switch for measuring vertical tilt and the speaker for the aversive tone.

In order to silently and accurately record the cumulative duration of slouching, a miniature elapsed time meter was arranged in series with the posture switch. The meter employed a capillary tube filled with two columns of mercury separated by a gap of electrolyte. When current passed through the meter, the electrolyte gap moved at a rate determined by the current flow. The speed of the timer was determined by the value of the fixed resistor in series with the time meter. Current was allowed to pass through the time meter only after the posture switch had been closed for three seconds.

All of the subjects who took part in this study slouched less when their slouching resulted in the punishing tone than when it did not have this effect. Each time the tone was disconnected as part of the research design, slouching increased. When the tone was reconnected, slouching again decreased. With two of the subjects the contingency was reversed, slouching terminating the tone rather than producing it. Both of these subjects exhibited an increase in slouching when the tone sounded and a decrease in slouching when the tone was inoperative. This effect serves to point up the effectiveness of the contingent stimuli.

The investigation by O'Brien and Azrin (1970) employed apparatus functionally identical to that used in the previous study, with the exception that slouching produced a vibrotactile stimulation to the subjects' shoulder instead of an auditory stimulus. The stimulus was produced by energizing a bone conductor, such as is used for patients with a hearing loss. This was attached to one of the shoulder straps of the harness so that it rested on the scapula.

Using eight nondisabled persons as subjects, the psychologists found that the tactile feedback decreased the percentage of time each subject spent slouching. The mean reduction in slouching was 35 percent. Thus, the vibrotactile stimulus reduced slouching when it was contingent upon it.

There is a major difference between this study and the one conducted by Azrin and his colleagues. While the latter investigation employed punishment for slouching and reinforcement in the form of escape for not slouching, the present research provided only informational feedback to the subjects regarding the status of their posture. (The authors do mention that there might have been some mild aversiveness to the vibratory stimulation.) The investigators did further research to determine the possible reasons for their results, and in a follow-up study found that it was the simple informational feedback which was effective in reducing the undesirable behavior.

It must be pointed out that all of the subjects in both studies were motivated towards improving their posture, and the authors state that in the absence of motivation, feedback alone most probably would not reduce the symptoms and, in fact, might exacerbate them. This is important for rehabilitation therapists to bear in mind should they wish to employ similar procedures with their disabled patients.

Muscle Strengthening

Upper extremity strength is essential for the performance of many activities, including transferring, propelling a wheelchair, and crutch walking, to name a few. Weakness of upper extremity strength can prevent an otherwise able patient from doing these tasks, and much time and effort must often be devoted to strengthening a patient's arms before he can progress on a physical therapy program.

Trotter and Inman (1968) hypothesized that a planned program of positive reinforcement would produce greater gains in upper extremity strengthening than would a physical therapy program which does not include systematic reinforcement.

They treated twelve paraplegic and twelve quadriplegic patients of both sexes. The patients were paired evenly for disability, sex, level of spinal cord lesion, hand dominance and muscle grade, and were matched as closely as possible for age and date of disability onset. Both the paraplegic and the quadriplegic patients had complete paralysis of the lower extremities. The quadriplegic patients had partial use of their arms and the paraplegics had full upper extremity function.

The members of each pair were assigned randomly to either an experimental or a control group. The mean age of the experimental group was 28.7 years, with a range of from sixteen to fifty-two years. The average age of the control group was 28.4 years, with a range of from sixteen to forty-five years.

Progressive resistance exercises were employed. The biceps muscles of the quadriplegics and the triceps muscles of the paraplegic patients were tested and the strength of these muscles was used as the dependent variable in the study. A ten repetition maximum, which is the maximal load a muscle can raise through the range of motion ten times, was determined each week for every subject.

Each pair of subjects was compaired during a four-week period. For biceps strengthening, the patients were seated in their wheelchairs, and precalibrated sandbags were placed over the forearm, just above the wrist. The sandbags were held in place by straps to prevent them from falling off as the arm was flexed at the elbow. The physical therapist or an assistant stabilized the patients' lower arms by placing a hand under their elbows. Substitution of shoulder muscles was prevented by the physical therapist placing an arm on the patients' shoulders. For the strengthening of triceps muscles, the patients lay in a supine position and held the sandbags in their hands. The therapist or assistant stabilized the arm as the patient extended it upward.

Once the control group subjects had learned the exercise program and could assume the proper position, they were permitted to perform the exercises independently or, in the case of the quadriplegic patients, with assistance from a nonprofessional staff member. While the usual conversation took place between the patients and the therapist or assistant, this neither was planned nor consistent. Reinforcement was not given for improved responding. Each week, a new ten repetition maximum was determined and recorded by the assistant, but this was not done in the presence of the subjects, nor was the increase discussed with them.

The subjects in the experimental group had the therapist relate the increases in lifting to them, verbally. These increases were also related to the appropriate rehabilitation goals, e.g. crutch walking, transferring, self-care and wheelchair mobility. After each ten repetitions, the patient was given a rest, and was praised and encouraged by the therapist. Each week, when the new ten repetition maximum was determined, the therapist reviewed the patient's record with him, stressing the increased amount of load, recording this in his presence, and applying the changes to present or future goals. Reinforcement, therefore, was both verbal and visual.

The data was analyzed by a mixed model analysis of variance. The obtained F ratio for the main treatment effect (Experimental versus Control) was 47.06, significant at the .001 level of confidence.

The average weight gain for the experimental group was 10.29 pounds, while the mean gain for the patients in the control group was only 2.40 pounds. This difference was not attributable to hand dominance, and most clearly was a direct consequence of the reinforcement procedures.

A question which arises after reading a study such as this concerns the matter of the delivery of reinforcement. Trotter and Inman used primarily verbal praise and feedback of performance. One may wonder what results would have been obtained had the entire procedure been automated, thus reducing the possibility of human error and/or inconsistency. This question is raised not as a criticism of the present investigation, but rather to suggest the possibility of more precise measures and reinforcement. Furthermore, with automation of procedures the therapist can be freed from spending much time with the subjects under consideration, and work with other patients or engage in other tasks.

With reference to the above study, for example, instead of using sandbags, standard metal weights can be employed, placed on a platform, which registers the total weight on a scale which is visible to the patient. The weights can be raised by means of a pulley system, the handle of the pulley held by the patient or attached to his extremity, with a switch mounted in the pulley shaft so that closure of the switch is activated by the weight touching it as it rises, and opening it as it descends. The switch can be connected to a light or an auditory signal so that each time the weight is raised to the level of the switch, the subject receives immediate reinforcement. The switch can be made movable within the pulley shaft, beginning at a level where only a slight raise of the weight will activate it, and progressing to higher levels as the patient gains in muscle strength and range of motion. A counter, also visible to the subject, can be wired to the switch so that each raise of the weight would activate it once. Thus, the patient can see how many times he was able to raise the weight to the desired height within each session. With such a system, the patient will know how much weight he is lifting, will be reinforced for responding at successive increases, and will be able to compare his performance from session to session without the need for much direct therapist involvement.

As an additional feature, each digit on the counter can be considered as a "point," and the patient can earn additional therapy time, canteen privileges, etc., in exchange for a predetermined number of points, similar to the operation of a token system.

This type of automation can be adapted to work with the lower extremities as well. Similar programming devices may be used with strengthening exercises, such as are performed on an Elgin table.

Reinforcement for ambulation activities can be electronically automated. For walking within parallel bars, a series of ribbon switches can be spaced at variable intervals along the platform and wired so that contact with a switch by a patient's foot activates a reinforcing stimulus such as a light, or a tone, or music, or a slide or film, or points on a counter. Patients who are learning to ambulate outside of the parallel bars can have ribbon switches placed under a long rubber mat or runner, or even directly on the floor. A more sophisticated approach might involve the use of "electric eyes" placed at intervals along the walkway, and each time a patient's leg crosses a beam the delivery of reinforcement would be triggered.

Programming of this nature requires an understanding of basic operant conditioning principles and familiarity with electronics, as well as knowledge of the fundamentals and techniques of physical therapy. Rehabilitation is a team effort, requiring the combined skills of various professionals, and this is one area for cooperation between the physical therapist and the psychologist.

* * * * * *

A second and somewhat different study dealing with the improvement of muscle strength was conducted by Fordyce, Sand, Trieschmann and Fowler (1971). The stated goal was an increase in the rate of lifting 12-pound dumbbells bilaterally, by a twenty-year-old, paraplegic woman who was on an exercise program for upper extremity strengthening.

In order to establish a baseline of performance, the patient was instructed to exercise at her own rate for as long as she was able to do so. No time limit was imposed on this activity, and her rate was observed and recorded for a two-minute exercise period. The patient completed sixteen cycles during the first minute, and six cycles in the second minute of work. It was believed, by the investigators, that the significant reduction in rate which occurred during the second minute was a result of fatigue. Therefore, her baseline was defined as sixteen cycles per minute and further exercise was limited to one-minute periods.

Then, rest was made contingent upon time. The patient was instructed to exercise for one minute, and then she could receive two minutes of rest. This procedure produced no increases over baseline measures.

Subsequently, rest was employed as a reinforcer contingent upon work, i.e. performing an increased number of cycles per minute of exercise. This had the result of raising the patient's rate to 27.3 cycles per minute, which was well above her previous maximum.

Reinforcing effort, rather than making reinforcement contingent upon the passage of time, has long been recognized as having desirous effects on performance. As many employers know, workers will produce more if they are paid for units of production than when they are paid for time spent on the job regardless of output. The above study demonstrates that the same principle apparently holds true for rehabilitation activities as well.

IMPROVING ENDURANCE

The same investigators (Fordyce, Sand, Trieschmann and Fowler, 1971) utilized both rest and attention as reinforcers to increase endurance in a middle-aged man who had pain in the knee and lower back as a consequence of degenerative joint disease.

The target behavior was designated as increased distance ridden on an unresisted, stationary bicycle. Performance was measured in tenths of a mile. Baseline data indicated that the patient rode an average of 1.4 miles per ten minutes of activity. Rest, attention in the form of praise from the therapist, and a publicly displayed graph showing performance were employed as reinforcers.

Riding trials were divided into two segments. Distance quotas were assigned, half of which were to be completed in each segment. When the patient completed the quota for the first segment, he was given a five-minute rest interval. If he did not complete the quota, one minute of rest was deducted for each tenth of a mile deficit. When he completed both segments and the total quota for the day, his therapist praised him appropriately and recorded his performance on the graph. The quotas were increased by two-tenths of a mile each day.

This technique had the result of increasing the patient's endurance on the bicycle exerciser by two-tenths of a mile per day. By the sixth day, he was riding 2.4 miles and the treatment goal had been achieved.

* * * * *

Although it is not possible to state precisely which contingent stimulus — rest, therapist praise, or the public display of progress — produced the desired effect, or which combination of stimuli was responsible for success, it is well known that attention from a therapist can mean a great deal to a patient. This is clearly demonstrated in some of the studies which have been described in this chapter (Fordyce, 1968; Fowler, Fordyce and Berni, 1969) and may have had a role in the success achieved by Trotter and Inman (1968). Therapists are aware of this but seldom use it to advantage and often tend to be attentive to their patients on a random, noncontingent basis, thus possibly reinforcing undesirable behaviors.

If a therapist observes that his or her interaction with a patient is important to him, she can use this skillfully as a reinforcer to improve the patient's functioning. It may appear "cruel" at times to withhold responses from a patient, but the long term benefits outweight the dissatisfaction of the moment.

INCREASING TOLERANCE FOR A BRACE

While an orthosis or a prosthesis may be prescribed and designed with the best interests of the patient in mind, it sometimes is found that the patient does not wear the device. This is true particularly for cumbersome apparatus, such as long-leg braces, but also is true of aids which require less effort to put on and take off. If it is deemed medically necessary or important for such a device to be worn, the failure or refusal of the patient to do so becomes a problem for concern.

Fowler, Fordyce and Berni (1969) treated a sixty-six-year-old woman who had experienced chronic back difficulties for more than twenty years. She had postmenopausal osteoporosis with multiple compression fractures of the spinal vertebrae. Although a back brace had been prescribed for her many years before, she had refused to wear it, claiming that it caused her great discomfort and restricted her motions. Prior to beginning the operant program, the longest period for which she had worn the brace during the previous two weeks had been thirty minutes.

The conditioning program required the patient to keep a record, in a small notebook, of each time she put on and took off the brace. For the first several days, the psychologist added up the total number of minutes she wore the brace, and these totals were recorded on a graph and placed on a bulletin board at the patient's bedside.

At the end of the first week of treatment all of the recording was turned over to the patient. Throughout the day, nurses and other staff members checked her graph and praised her for increased tolerance of the brace. If there were declines in tolerance they made no comment at all. Within less than four weeks after the initiation of the reinforcement procedure, the patient was discharged.

The effect of the program was that at discharge time the patient was wearing the back brace approximately thirty-three hours per week. When she left the hospital she was given a supply of graph paper, and was requested to continue her recording. She returned to the hospital for a brief check, once per week, and at this time the psychologists transferred her week's record to a permanent record. During a seven-and one-half week out-patient follow-up period she wore the brace for between thirty-two and thirty-seven hours per week. She was very proud of her records and spontaneously displayed them to anyone who evidenced interest. Figure 3-7 illustrates this patient's progress.

There are two points which are interesting to discuss in relation to this study. One concerns the phenomenon of social reinforcement. Social reinforcement, in the form of attention and/or praise from persons in the environment can exert very powerful influences on an individual's behavior. A common example of this is the obese person who loses a significant amount of weight and consequently is praised by her family and friends, frequently told

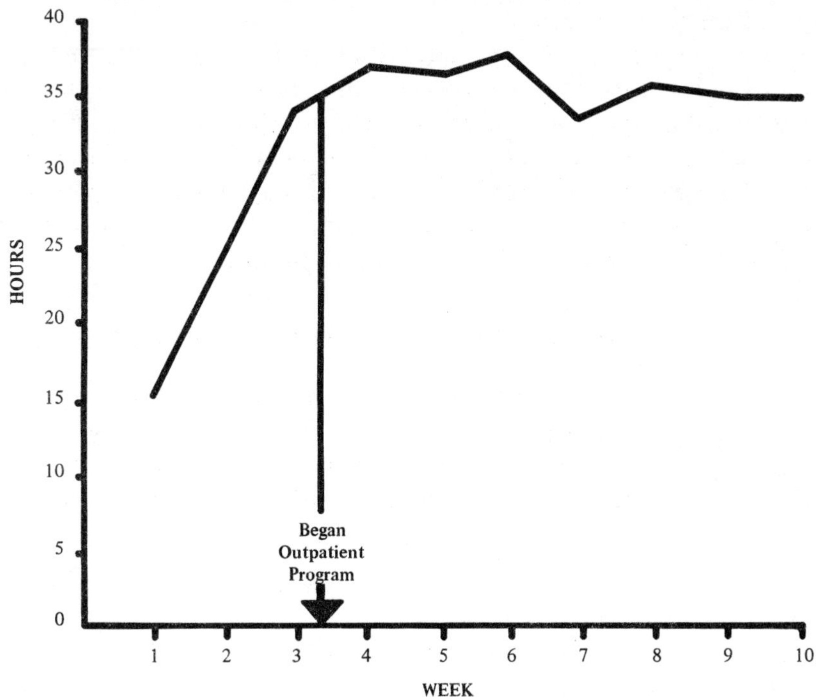

Figure 3-7 Progress in wearing a back brace. From Fowler, R. S., Fordyce, W. E. and Berni, Rosemarian: Operant conditioning in chronic illness. *Am J Nurs, June*:1226, 1969.

Reproduced with the permission of the senior author and the *American Journal of Nursing*. Copyright June, 1969, The American Journal of Nursing Company.

how nice she looks, becomes able to wear stylish clothing and is complimented on this, and so on. These are the kinds of reinforcers that "take over" once the person leaves the laboratory or the institutional environment where the contingencies are experimentally controlled.

The patient in the case just presented received praise from hospital staff members for increased tolerance of the back brace, and it is highly probable that she also received similar reinforcement from her family upon her return home. In fact, she actually sought out such reinforcement from others, as evidenced by her readiness to show her progress records to anyone who expressed an interest in them.

A second feature of this study which is of interest is the involvement of the patient in her own conditioning program. After the first few days she was made responsible for the maintenance of her own records and graphs. People often become much more motivated towards achievement when they share in their program and are integrally involved in it than when something is done to them without their active and willing participation.

CONTROLLING HEAD MOVEMENTS

Correct body and head position often are important prerequisites for a physical therapy program. When there are problems in this area of motor functioning, considerable time may have to be devoted to correcting the dysfunction before a full rehabilitation program can be prescribed.

This was the case with a sixteen-year-old girl treated by Grove (1970). Her medical diagnosis was one of spastic quadriplegia with choreo-athetosis, secondary to encephalopathy. The patient's physical therapist had observed that she spent a considerable proportion of her time with her head held in other than an erect or extended position. The therapist identified control of head positioning as a beginning objective of the patient's rehabilitation program.

A cloth collar was fitted around the patient's neck so that it did not interfere with normal head movements. Four mercury switches were attached to this collar and wired in sequence so that any movement of the patient's head away from the desired position would open the contacts on one of the switches and break the circuit. Scheduling was accomplished by standard programming apparatus. Data were recorded on electrical impulse counters and elapsed time meters. The onset of a small transistor radio, which served as a reinforcer, was also controlled by the programming equipment.

The patient was seen during thirty-minute therapy sessions, two or three times per day, with a brief interval between sessions.

The study was conducted in a curtained area of the physical therapy treatment room. Reliability of the measures taken by the switches was confirmed by four independent observers. Reliability between the switches and the judgement of the observers was between 85 percent and 90 percent, with a mean of 88 percent.

During the baseline phase, a record was obtained of the amount of time which the patient's head was maintained in the desired position of extension. There was no reinforcement given for correct behavior during this time.

In Phase II, reinforcement in the form of the onset of the transistor radio was made contingent upon holding the head in the correct position.

In Phase III, causality was demonstrated by delivering reinforcement for every head position other than the desired one.

Reinforcement contingent upon the correct response was reinstated in Phase IV.

Phase V consisted of removing all reinforcement to determine whether extinction of the desired head position would occur.

In Phase VI, all of the variables were maintained, but the radio was kept on during the entire thirty-minute session regardless of head position.

Phase VII reestablished the contingency of the onset of the radio for proper head positioning.

Figure 3-8 shows the percentage of time that the patient held her head in the proper position during each thirty-minute session of the experiment.

During the baseline phase she held her head correctly an average of 8 percent of the total time. During Phase II, the first reinforcement period, this percentage varied between 88 percent and 99 percent, with a mean of 94 percent for six sessions. In Phase III, reinforcement for all other head positions but the correct one resulted in a decline in responding to three percent, but reestablishment of the reinforcement contingency raised it to a mean of 91 percent. Extinction, in Phase V, produced erratic behavior, and percentages varied between zero and 72 percent, with a mean of 4.75 percent over the last four sessions. In Phase VI, when the radio was continuously on, the percent of correct head positioning was 27 percent. The final phase of the study,

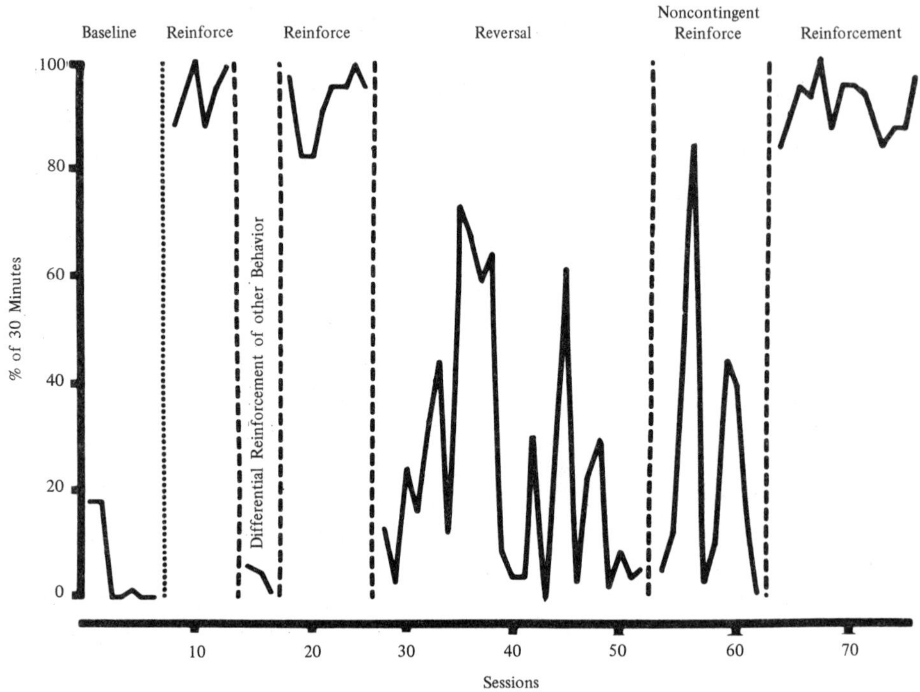

Figure 3-8 Head position (extension). From Grove, D. N.: Application of behavioral technology to physical therapy. Paper presented at the Annual Convention of the American Psychological Association, Miami Beach, 1970.

Reproduced with the permission of the author and the American Psychological Association.

when onset of the radio was made contingent upon desired behavior once again, resulted in a mean of 91 percent correct responding for 14 sessions. There was no doubt that the scheduled reinforcement produced the desired change in behavior and that environmental contingencies alone did not effect responding in the proper direction.

As Grove's work demonstrates, it is highly important to introduce a step in the procedure where the reinforcement contingencies are reversed, as was done in Phase III, and to have an extinction period. Only by doing so can the investigator attribute causality to his techniques and be able to state with reasonable certainty that it was the reinforcement contingency which resulted in the desired effects.

REFERENCES

Azrin, N., Rubin, H., O'Brien, F., Ayllon, T., and Roll D.: Behavioral engineering: Postural control by a portable operant apparatus. *J Appl Behav Anal, 1*:99, 1968.

Di Scipio, W. J. and Feldman, M. C.: Combined behavior therapy and physical therapy in the treatment of a fear of walking. *J Behav Ther Exp Psychiat, 2*:151, 1971.

Fordyce, W. E.: The learning model and psychology's role in medical rehabilitation. Paper presented at the Annual Convention of the American Psychological Association, San Francisco, 1968.

Fordyce, W. E., Sand, Patricia L., Trieschmann, Roberta B. and Fowler, R. S.: Behavioral systems analyzed. *J Rehabil, 37*:29, 1971.

Fowler, R. S., Fordyce, W. E. and Berni, Rosemarian: Operant conditioning in chronic illness. *Am J Nurs, June*:1226, 1969.

Goodkin, R.: Case studies in behavioral research in rehabilitation. *Percept Mot Skills, 23*:171, 1966.

Grove, D. N.: Application of behavioral technology to physical therapy. Paper presented at the Annual Convention of the American Psychological Association, Miami Beach, 1970.

Horner, R. D.: Establishing use of crutches by a mentally retarded spina bifida child. *J Appl Behav Anal, 4*:183, 1971.

Ince, L. P.: Behavior modification in a rehabilitation service setting. Paper presented at the Annual Convention of the American Psychological Association, San Francisco, 1968.

Ince, L. P.: *The Rehabilitation Medicine Services.* Springfield, Thomas, 1974.

Meyerson, L., Kerr, Nancy and Michael, J.: Behavior modification in rehabilitation. In Bijou, S. W. and Baer, D. M. (Eds): *Child Development: Readings in Experimental Analysis.* New York: Appleton-Century-Crofts, 1967.

O'Brien, F. and Azrin, N. H.: Behavior engineering: Control of posture by informational feedback. *J Appl Behav Anal, 3*:235, 1970.

Rachman, S.: The role of muscular relaxation in desensitization therapy. *Behav Res Ther, 6*:159, 1968.

Trotter, Ann B. and Inman, D. A.: The use of positive reinforcement in physical therapy. *J Am Phys Ther Assoc, 48*:347, 1968.

Chapter Four

CONDITIONING TECHNIQUES IN OCCUPATIONAL THERAPY

THERE IS OFTEN an overlapping of function between occupational therapy and physical therapy. For example, both disciplines may work towards increasing strength in a patient's arms, the physical therapist doing so in order to enable the patient to ambulate with crutches, the occupational therapist to permit him to perform the necessary activities of daily living (see Ince, 1974). However, it is typically the case that the physical therapist works primarily with a patient's lower extremities, while the occupational therapist concentrates on upper extremity function. For purposes of clarity and convenience, therefore, this chapter focuses on the latter activities.

THE EVALUATION

Regardless of the type of rehabilitation institution in which one works, or the disability one is planning to treat, or the form of therapy one is considering to utilize in the treatment procedure, prior to any therapeutic endeavor an evaluation must be made of the limitations, capabilities and potential of the involved patient.

A unique method for evaluating upper extremity skills has been developed by Friedlander, using an automated system known as PLAYTEST®. The PLAYTEST system consists of a series of consoles, each composed of an array of panels providing for a variety of upper extremity tasks such as pushing a disc, turning a knob, pulling a lever, moving a ring, operating a light switch, pulling a drawer knob, grasping a handle, and the like. Correct manipulation results in the delivery of reinforcement, in the form of door chimes, music, colored lights, and similar stimuli. Lamps, mounted above or behind each manipulandum, signal the subject regarding which response will produce reinforcement. The manipulanda can be programmed to operate individually, sequentially, or in various combinations. The apparatus and the contingencies are automatically programmed and timed. The system also records the subject's performance in terms of the number and cumulative duration of responses. It is able to measure finger flexion and extension, wrist pronation and supination, arm flexion and extension, pinch, grasp, integrated functions, coordination, and other upper extremity function variables in a precise and reliable manner. Furthermore, it offers a relatively high repetition of similar tasks, thereby facilitating skill development.

Friedlander and his associates (Friedlander, Gencheff, Moore and Nelson, 1969) employed the automated apparatus with twenty-two patients whose ages ranged from five to twenty years. The patients' diagnoses included spastic hemiplegia, spastic quadriplegia, athetosis, post-traumatic diffuse, central nervous system dysfunction, spastic cerebral palsy, upper extremity amputation, and mixed cerebral palsy. All of the patients were severely mentally retarded in addition to their physical disabilities.

All of the sessions were conducted by an occupational therapist. Individual sessions varied in length from a duration of one minute to fifteen minutes, with a modal session duration of approximately twelve minutes. The therapist selected the program for each day, supervised the patients' activities during the sessions, and recorded the data.

The first task, a visual-motor tracking task, required the patient to reach out and touch a red disc inset in each of six panels on the console, when the disc was illuminated from behind by a bright red signal lamp. The timing and the order of activation of each signal lamp was automatically regulated. The patient's correct responses were reinforced with chimes and music. During most of the sessions, the cue lights shifted position every six seconds, sometimes in ordered sequence from left to right and sometimes in random order. Simpler presentations were employed when the patients were first learning the task.

The regularity of performance on this task can be seen by examination of Table 4-I, which represents the performance of some of the patients. The upper section of the table presents the

Tasks	*October*	*November*	*December*
Group Means	(15)	(24)	(14)
right hand responses	65.0 secs.	83.6 secs.	90.2 secs.
left hand responses	52.7	57.5	68.2
ordered sequence	65.2	74.2	84.1
random sequence	56.5	72.2	76.0
Mean of means	59.9	71.9	79.6
Individual Means	(3)	(6)	(5)
right hand responses	54.	88.	96.
left hand responses	38.	70.	78.
ordered sequence	50.	83.	92.
random sequence	42.	81.	83.
Mean of means	46.0	80.5	87.3

*Note that right hand response means are uniformly higher than left hand means, and ordered sequence means are uniformly higher than random sequence means (see text).

Table 4-I Correct time on target in visual motor tracking tasks. From Friedlander, B. Z., Gencheff, T., Moore, Marie and Nelson, Kay: Automated exercise procedures in evaluation and rehabilitation of upper extremity motor skills with seriously disabled institutional retardates. Paper presented at the Annual Convention of the American Association on Mental Deficiency, San Francisco, 1969.

Reproduced with the permission of the senior author.

summary means for four boys (Mean C.A.=7.5 years, Mean M.A.=2.0 years) who were tested over a three-month period on four subtasks. The subtasks called for performing the tracking in ordered sequence and in randomized sequence, with both the left hand and the right hand. The lower portion of the table presents the same data for one representative member of the group. The figures in parentheses refer to the number of sessions.

On each subtask, and for overall performance, there is a highly systematic upward progression over the three-month period. There are no inversions, and performance is regular, despite the fact that there was an interruption in the program from early November to mid-December. In fact, the December scores show further increment, as if there had been concentrated practice. It also can be seen that all right-handed performance measures are higher than all left-handed measures, and that the patients performed better on tasks of ordered presentation than they did on the more difficult randomly sequenced presentations.

The second task was a manual guidance and control activity, requiring the patient to move a ring along a rod without letting the ring come into contact with the rod. Rods of different lengths and varied configurations necessitated that the patient make different kinds of movements at the wrist, elbow and shoulder. Rings of varying diameters posed a number of levels of difficulty.

While the ring was not touching the rod, the patient performing the task was continuously reinforced with pleasing music. When the ring contacted the rod, the music was replaced by an aversive, piercing whine from a sound alarm. The PLAYTEST system kept a record of the frequency and the duration of errors (ring-rod contacts), the total time of the ring in transit along the rod, and the number of transits which the patient made with the ring from one end of the rod to the other. The sessions typically consisted of a series of two-minute trials with various rods and rings.

Figure 4-I is the record of a ten-year-old boy with mixed cerebral palsy and quadriplegia. The solid lines represent productivity and the broken lines denote the error scores. When he was using his left hand, errors decreased as transit productivity increased. With his right hand, however, even slight increases in productivity resulted in a marked increase in errors.

The apparatus and methodology used in this study were demonstrably effective in producing extensive runs of measurable performance from a patient group whose performance usually is considered to be quite limited. It is important to realize that not only can such procedures be employed to evaluate the potential performance of the disabled but, because of their practical features, have direct relevance for therapy and training.

REDUCING SPASTICITY

A significant problem observed in many rehabilitation

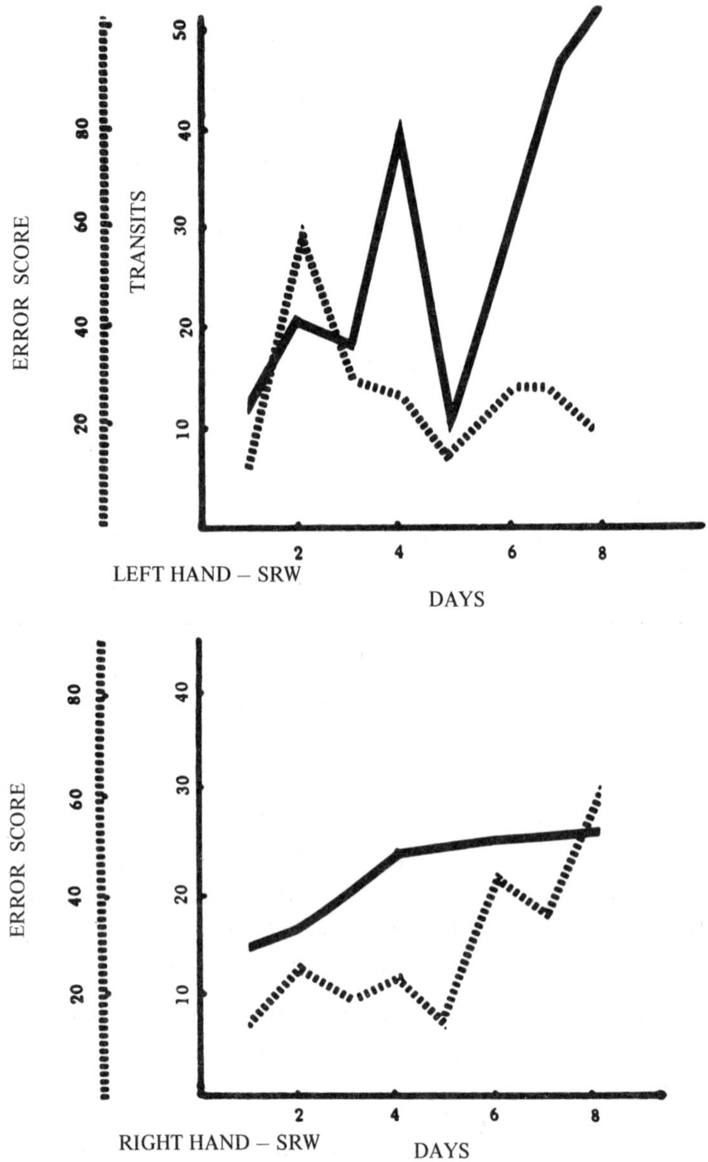

Figure 4-1 Left and right hand performance by a ten-year-old boy with mixed CP quadriplegia on a manual guidance and control task using a two-inch ring on a large, parabolic, wicket-shaped rod. From Friedlander, B. Z., Gencheff, T., Moore, Marie and Nelson, Kay: Automated exercise procedures in evaluation and rehabilitation of upper extremity motor skills with seriously disabled institutional retardates. Paper presented at the Annual Convention of the American Association on Mental Deficiency, San Francisco, 1969.

Reproduced with the permission of the senior author.

patients, particularly those with some form of paralysis, is muscle spasticity. When spasticity is severe, it can prevent a patient from using his affected body part in a functional manner, and often from moving the part at all. An occupational therapy program may have to be very limited in its goals unless the spasticity is relieved and, hence, this becomes a serious problem to deal with.

A conditioning procedure was employed to reduce hand spasticity by Block, Forster, Ma, Wietfeldt and Murase (1971). They treated six patients with left hemiplegia and seven with right hemiplegia. The patients ranged in age from twelve to sixty-six years, and the durations of their disabilities varied between one month and eleven years. The specific goal of the study was the promotion of volitional control of the relaxation of the spastic muscles, particularly those of the thumb and index finger, which are of primary importance in basic hand functions. One of the patients had treatment directed at a dorsiflexed wrist. All of the patients exhibited marked spasticity, and none had shown any improvement with conventional therapy methods. The prognosis for achieving a functional hand was considered to be poor for most of the patients.

The patient's affected arm was placed on a long projecting board and restrained with rubber straps. A box was placed before the patient, containing electronic apparatus which performed, in a more sophisticated way, the functions of a spring and mechanical meter linkage system. A string was projected through a hole in the box, and this was attached to the patient's finger tip. A curtain obscured the patient's view of the apparatus, but permitted him to see a meter which displayed the extension movement of his finger. The string applied a constant, adjustable force to the finger. This force acted to extend the finger against an opposing spastic flexor muscle. Such a movement of the involved digit, and thus of the string, was linked to the needle of the meter so that amplification was obtained. By doing this, even a slight finger movement of only one millimeter could result in a large needle deflection. A polygraph recorded all finger movements during each thirty minute experimental session.

The patient was instructed to move the needle of the meter

between zero and full scale as rapidly and as frequently as possible. Flexion usually is rapid, and the patient spends the majority of time learning to relax the spastic flexors and allow the finger to be pulled into extension. During his neural searching, if the patient happened to activate a circuit which reduced spasticity even slightly and briefly, the force exerted on the finger tip served to create an actual movement of the finger which was amplified and displayed as a large, unambiguous deflection on the meter. This feedback to the patient served as a reinforcer for desired responding.

Ten of the thirteen subjects, or 77 percent, showed a significant, progressive improvement in learning to control their spasticity. The causal effect of the reinforcement was demonstrated, since a control group of five patients who received only the extensor force but not the meter feedback did not learn the response as did the experimental group.

Although the investigation was designed only to reduce spasticity and not to improve function, some of the patients did exhibit functional gains, performing tasks such as picking up and carrying objects and bags with handles, writing, eating, and partially dressing.

As the investigators noted, it appears that control of muscle spasticity can be learned, at least to some extent. Importantly, methods such as those employed in this research can routinely be incorporated into the treatment program of patients with severe, chronic spasticity so that they may become amenable to further occupational therapy for improvement of function.

* * * * *

Sachs and Mayhall (1971) used punishment to reduce the general spasms of a twenty-year-old, cerebral palsied man. The patient displayed a variety of involuntary motor behaviors, including uncoordinated and undirected movements of his head trunk and extremities.

The patient and an investigator sat in a small room facing each other, approximately four feet apart, and engaged in conversation during thirty minute sessions. The first four sessions constituted the baseline period, during which three types of spastic movements were identified and recorded. These were as follows:

1. Gross head movements — movements of the head while the patient was speaking, which resulted in loss of eye contact for a minimum time of two seconds;
2. Spasms — irrelevant movements of the arms, legs or trunk;
3. Combination behaviors — the temporal joint occurrence of gross head movements and spasms.

The programming and recording apparatus were located in an adjoining room and were not viewable by the patient. The patient had electrodes attached to the second and third fingers of his preferred hand. The investigator held a small box which had three buttons mounted on it, each button corresponding to a different undesirable behavior, as identified during the baseline phase.

During the baseline period, the depression of a button only counted the occurrence of a response. During the subsequent aversive conditioning sessions, the depression of a button additionally delivered a .75-second, 2.5 milliampere Direct Current (ma DC) shock to the patient's fingers. This punishment procedure continued for eight sessions.

Figure 4-2 presents the data. The first four sessions indicate the baseline period. During this phase, the frequency of gross movements varied between 35 and 54. Spasms ranged between 6 and 21, and cumulative behaviors varied from three to six. The total number of undesirable behaviors ranged between 45 and 82.

When the punishment contingency was introduced, it resulted in an immediate reduction of gross head movements and a gradual decline in spasms. During the final four sessions of the conditioning phase, the range of gross head movements was between 2 and 13, the range for spasms was from one to three, and combination behaviors had a zero rate of occurrence.

The results obtained in this study imply that for the patient involved, spastic behavior was the consequence of both cerebral dysfunction and learning. Successful treatment does not require the knowledge of how or why the learning occurred, although, as the authors note, concepts such as escape or avoidance learning or secondary gain may provide the framework for neurologically

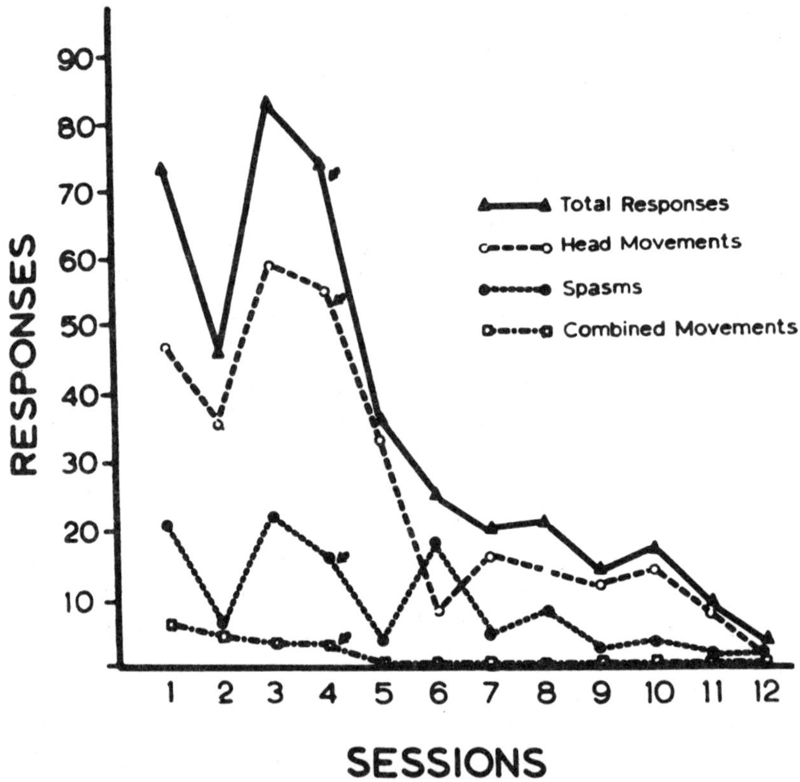

Figure 4-2 Response rate of head movement, spasms, combined movements and total responses per session of a twenty-year-old cerebral palsied male. From Sachs, D. A. and Mayhall, B.: Behavioral control of spasms using aversive conditioning with a cerebral palsied adult. *J Nerv Ment Dis, 152*:362, 1971.

Reproduced with the permission of the senior author and the *Journal of Nervous and Mental Disease*. Copyright 1971, the Williams and Wilkins, Co., Baltimore, Maryland.

produced behaviors to develop learned components and increase in frequency.

It cannot conclusively be stated that techniques such as those employed by Sachs and Mayhall will always be successful in reducing the spasticity of patients with cerebral palsy. However, when a patient's behavior does appear to be under the control of external stimuli and thus at least partially learned, a behavioral approach may prove highly fruitful.

UPPER EXTREMITY MOVEMENT

Gross Movements

While function is the ultimate goal in occupational therapy, movement is, of course, the necessary prerequisite. In 1949, Fuller conditioned an eighteen-year-old "vegetative idiot" to move his arms, a behavior which he had never previously performed. In 1968, Rice, McDaniel and Denney used a similar procedure with a six-year-old boy.

The patient was mentally retarded, functioning at the level of a three-month-old infant. He was diagnosed as having severe cerebral palsy, secondary to perinatal anoxia. The only movements which he was able to control voluntarily were those of the eyes and face. When he attempted to assist in being picked up or dressed, the result was a spastic rigidity of his entire body.

The child was placed in a crib resembling a traction bed. A red darning hoop was suspended from a cross-bar above the bed and lowered to a height of approximately one foot above the child's right hand. A twenty-minute baseline period was used to observe the patient and record any unelicited movements toward the hoop. While spontaneous movement did occur, he did not touch the hoop during this period.

Next, the desired response of touching the hoop was shaped by successive approximations. The patient first was reinforced for movement of the right arm in any direction; a spoonful of ice cream served as the reinforcer. Once he was moving his arm at a satisfactory rate, only those movements which were made in the general direction of the darning hoop were reinforced. Gradually, the experimenters became more stringent in their requirement of how close his arm or hand had to come to the hoop for reinforcement to be given until, finally, only actually touching the hoop was reinforced.

Eventually, it became possible to place the patient's responding on an FR15 reinforcement schedule and, at one point he touched the hoop more than 700 times during a single forty-five minute period.

This study, like the one by Fuller, illustrates that low intelligence is not necessarily a deterrant when trying to instate movement. Neither, apparently, is age, verbal ability, or motivation. Rice et al. did not continue their investigation further, and so it remains speculative as to whether the child could have learned to use his arm in a functional manner. However, since the conditioned response was a relatively precise one, and not merely an increase in the patient's general level of activity, this possibility may be considered.

* * * * *

Ince (1969) employed escape and avoidance conditioning techniques in an effort to directly influence the motor return in the involved upper extremities of hemiplegic patients.

Two male patients, aged forty-one and fifty-eight years, and one female patient aged sixty-seven years, all with left hemiplegia resulting from a cerebrovascular accident were the subjects. The males had sustained their strokes nine and ten months, respectively, prior to the study, and the female patient had suffered her stroke six months before her participation in the experiment.

All subjects received a neurological examination before the research was initiated, and all were judged to have nonfunctional left upper extremities. The male patients both graded *zero* on all muscle tests, and both had marked spasticity of the left arm. The female subject was graded *trace* for shoulder elevator and rotator muscles, and *zero* for shoulder abductor, flexor and extensor muscles.

Elbow flexion was selected as the response to condition since it is a relatively gross and simple behavior, and is easier than finer motor movements for the hemiplegic patient to execute.

A baseline phase of fifty sessions of fifteen minutes duration each revealed that none of the patients was able to voluntarily perform a single elbow flexion response. The patients then were assigned randomly to either an escape or an avoidance condition. The female patient, referred to hereafter as F-1, and one male patient, hereafter called M-1, received escape conditioning. The other male subject, M-2, was treated with avoidance conditioning techniques.

In both experimental conditions, the forearm of the subject's nonplegic upper extremity was immobilized by taping it to the arm of the wheelchair. Two copper electrodes were attached to this forearm, one on the dorsal and one on the ventral surfaces. The forearm was rubbed lightly with sandpaper to decrease skin resistance, and the electrodes were sheathed in thin canvas which had been soaked in a saline solution to increase conductivity. The paralyzed upper extremity was positioned on a wooden board, which was clamped to the other arm of the wheelchair by a small vise. This arm remained free to move. Attached to the board by a wing nut was a wooden arm which could be raised or lowered to any desired height. A microswitch was mounted at the distal end of the wooden arm.

In the escape condition, the subject received an electric shock to the forearm of the nonplegic upper extremity, which could be terminated only by a flexion response of the plegic arm, so that the hand contacted the microswitch which turned off the current. If the subject did not make the appropriate response within ten seconds following the onset of the shock, the shock was terminated automatically and remained off for five seconds.

In the avoidance situation, a brief "click" was presented five seconds before the onset of the shock. A flexion response of the paralyzed upper extremity, occurring between the click and the shock, postponed the onset of the shock for ten seconds.

All subjects received a current intensity which varied between 2.5 and 3.5 ma, delivered from a standard chronaxie apparatus (see Ince, 1974).

The subjects were begun at a criterion of five degrees of elbow flexion. That is, the wooden arm with the microswitch was positioned so that it required a flexion response of five degrees by the plegic arm for the hand to contact the switch, thus terminating or postponing the shock. If a subject was able to make the desired response ten times in succession, the wooden arm was raised by five degrees until the criterion of ten consecutive responses had been made at that level, and was raised thereafter in steps of five degrees. When a subject could not meet the initial criterion, the wooden arm was lowered to a position where responding could occur and then was advanced from that level. If no notable increases in responding, from baseline level were observed within twenty experimental sessions, the procedure was terminated. Experimental sessions were of approximately fifteen minutes duration.

Neither M-1 nor M-2 were able to make any remarkable elbow flexion responses within twenty sessions, and their participation in the study was concluded.

Sessions	Trials	Mean Degrees Flexion	Frequency Response Emitted	Current Level (In mA)
1	60	0	—	2.5
2	60	11.5	6	2.5
3	60	23	5	3.1
4	45	39	9	2.5
5	40	30	14	3.0
6	40	35	19	3.2
7	40	50	12	3.2
8	30	40	7	3.2
9	60	45	10	3.1
10	100	45	8	3.1
11	100	40	4	3.2
12	100	40	5	3.2
13	100	40	5	3.2
14	100	60	4	3.2
15	100	50	4	3.0
16	100	60	3	3.0
17	100	70	4	3.1
18	100	70	4	3.0
19	100	70	5	3.0
20	100	60	7	3.0
21	100	70	6	3.0
22	100	50	7	3.0
23	100	45	6	3.0
24	100	40	6	3.2
25	100	45	7	3.2

Table 4-II Mean responses of patient F-1 per experimental session. From Ince, L. P.: Escape and avoidance conditioning of responses in the plegic arm of stroke patients: A preliminary study. *Psychon Sci, 16*:49, 1969.

Reproduced with the permission of *Psychonomic Science*.

The data for F-1, who did show significant changes, are presented in Table 4-II. It can be seen that during the second session this patient averaged 11.5 degrees of elbow flexion over sixty trials. She progressed to a mean of 70 degrees of flexion, and her responses varied between a mean of 40 degrees and a mean of 70 degrees for the last nineteen sessions. While there were some shoulder elevations as well as elbow flexions in her responses, they were primarily true, critical responses.

A neurological examination was conducted upon conclusion of the study and the following changes were noted: shoulder elevator muscles graded *fair-minus;* shoulder abductor muscles graded *trace-poor-minus;* shoulder rotator, flexor and extensor muscles graded *trace;* and elbow flexor muscles graded *trace.* All muscle grades showed improvement over baseline status.

* * * * *

A similar study was conducted by Halberstam, Zaretsky, Brucker and Guttman (1971) who worked with elderly (mean age=64.66 years), brain-damaged and nonbrain-damaged patients.

The subjects were divided into four groups of ten patients each. There was one group of brain-damaged patients with aphasia, one group of brain-damaged patients without aphasia, and two groups of nonbrain-damaged patients consisting of amputees, arthritics, and so on. In addition, five brain-damaged patients with aphasia, and five brain-damaged patients without aphasia were seen in repeated conditioning sessions for three weeks. The brain-damaged subjects were all patients who had hemiplegia, with both right- and left-sided involvement, secondary to cerebrovascular accidents. All subjects were administered a speech and hearing evaluation for purposes of assignment to the experimental groups, and all subjects also received a neurological examination to determine brain damage, spasticity, and experimental group assignment.

The subjects had electrodes placed one inch apart on the dorsal surface of the nonaffected upper extremity, midway between the wrist and the elbow. Electrode jelly was used to enhance conduction. The conditioning apparatus consisted of one metal plate attached to a horizontally movable board, and another metal plate fixed to a vertically movable board. Both boards were marked off in three-inch intervals, and could be moved to a maximum of one foot. Each of the plates was wired so that when a plate was touched by a subject it would break the conditioning stimulus (CS) and the unconditioned stimulus (UCS) circuits. The subject's plegic upper extremity rested on an armrest of the wheelchair.

There were two conditioning stimuli. The auditory stimulus consisted of a 1000 cps tone of 40 db, presented through a speaker which was located directly behind the subject's head. The visual stimulus was a one-inch diameter disc, illuminated by a six-watt incandescent bulb placed 30 inches before the subject. The unconditioned stimulus was electric shock, delivered to the nonplegic arm, at 25 volts and less than two ma, each subject selecting the shock value which he considered "mildly uncomfortable" for himself.

Prior to the actual conditioning sessions, each subject was seen during a baseline period to determine his maximal performance level for both vertical and horizontal arm movements. There were twenty pretest trials administered for each plane of movements. During this phase of the study, the experimenter simply said, "Go," and the subject was required to reach either the horizontal or the vertical plate, which were set at distances of three, six, nine, and twelve inches for him.

Following the baseline period, the electrodes were affixed to the patient's nonplegic upper extremity, the patient selected his shock tolerance level, and the conditioning procedure began. The subjects were informed that they would hear a tone or see a light, and receive shock during the experiment, and that they could avoid the shock by making an appropriate response. The CS-UCS interval was of five seconds duration, with a twenty-second intertrial interval. The duration of the UCS was two seconds. When the subject responded within the five-second CS-UCS interval, the response was recorded as an avoidance response. When the subject moved his arm correctly during the two-second UCS period, it was recorded as an escape response.

In the horizontal condition, the subjects were required to move their paralyzed arm for a distance of 3, 6, 9 and 12 inches in a horizontal direction. In the vertical condition, they had to raise their entire arm for the same distances. Twenty trials were administered at each distance; if a subject failed to respond at any distance for ten consecutive trials, the series was terminated for him. When a subject reached his maximum performance level, twenty extinction trials were conducted with the CS presented alone. This was followed by twenty post-test trials which were identical to the pretest condition of the study.

In the first phase of the experiment, two groups of nonbrain-damaged patients were administered the CS-UCS conditioning, one group receiving the light stimulus as the CS and the other group receiving the tone. In the second phase, three experimental groups (ten brain-damaged patients with aphasia, ten brain-damaged patients without aphasia, and ten nonbrain-damaged patients) received the same procedure, with sound alone as the CS.

Then, the five most severely brain-damaged patients with aphasia, and the five most severely brain-damaged nonaphasic patients were given two additional sessions of both the horizontal and the vertical conditioning tasks. These sessions were conducted at one-week intervals. After these sessions, forty extinction trials were conducted, followed by a final posttest.

Several interesting results were obtained from this research. *First,* it was demonstrated that sound is a more effective conditioning stimulus for both vertical and horizontal movements, with regard to latency of responding and mean number of appropriate responses.

Second, while there were no statistically significant differences in speed of responding between nonbrain-damaged and brain-damaged subjects at distances of 3 and 6 inches, the nonbrain-damaged subjects exhibited a trend towards shorter latencies, and a significant difference between the groups was found at both the 9-inch and 12-inch distances.

Third, there were no significant differences in speed of responding between subjects who had aphasia and subjects who did not.

Fourth, the effects of the conditioning on response latencies for all subjects, regardless of experimental group, were greater for responses made in the vertical direction than for horizontal responses.

Fifth, there was a marked decrease in response time, particularly among the aphasic brain-damaged subjects from pretest to posttest.

Sixth, the brain-damaged group with aphasia showed considerably less mean general improvement than did the non-aphasic brain-damaged group. For the former, the mean percent improvement was 33 percent in the horizontal direction and 24 percent in the vertical direction, while for the latter, the respective figures were 46 percent and 40 percent.

Seventh, for both directional planes, the brain-damaged subjects with aphasia showed an increasing percentage of improvement in speed of responding as the number of conditioning sessions increased. While a similar trend emerged for the non-aphasic, brain-damaged subjects, this trend was not consistent for those subjects. The data are presented in Table 4-III.

Response distance and conditioning session	Horizontal, % Without speech impairment	With speech impairment	Vertical, % Without speech impairment	With speech impairment
3 inches				
First session	55.0	33.0	15.0	33.0
Third session	59.0	56.0	23.0	33.0
6 inches				
First session	61.0	6.0	52.0	44.0
Third session	65.0	24.0	60.0	62.0
9 inches				
First session	53.0	30.0	43.0	20.0
Third session	53.0	50.0	39.0	57.0
12 inches				
First session	5.0	28.0	23.0	43.0
Third session	19.0	52.0	9.0	59.0
Overall				
First session	44.0	24.0	33.0	35.0
Third session	49.0	46.0	33.0	53.0

Table 4-III Mean percentage improvement in speed of response (N = 5 brain-damaged subjects in each group). From Halberstam, J. L., Zaretsky, H. H., Brucker, B. S. and Guttman, Andrea: Avoidance conditioning of motor responses in elderly brain damaged patients. *Arch Phys Med Rehabil, 52*:318, 1971.

Reproduced with the permission of the senior author and the *Archives of Physical Medicine and Rehabilitation.*

In the horizontal direction, both brain-damaged groups made approximately 75 percent correct responses at the 3-inch and 6-inch distances. When the distance was increased to 9 and 12-inches, only three of the five subjects in each group were able to make 50 percent correct responses during the first conditioning session. As the conditioning sessions continued, all subjects became able to respond correctly at all distances. At the 3-inch and 6-inch distances, they made nearly 100 percent correct responses. At the 9-inch distance, the subjects made 90 percent correct responses. Responding was 60 percent correct at the 12-inch distance. The results for responding in the vertical plane followed the same general pattern.

Last, all groups failed to extinguish their conditioned responses and continued to maintain their respective performance levels during the extinction phase of the experiment.

There are certain similarities between the study conducted by Ince and the later one of Halberstam and his colleagues. Both used escape and avoidance conditioning techniques; both worked with subjects who were brain-damaged and hemiplegic, both achieved results with elderly patients, and with patients who had suffered strokes several months prior to experimentation; and both treated responses which have direct relevance for rehabilitation, i.e. movement of the upper extremity.

Ince concluded that it is possible to condition motor return in hemiplegics as late as six months following the initial brain insult. Halberstam et al. summarized by stating that such procedures could prove a valuable adjunct to rehabilitation therapy. Taken together, these investigations illustrate the point that even among elderly, brain-damaged patients who have been hemiplegic for a relatively long period of time, it is possible to restore motor ability, perhaps to the extent that function can be returned to the disabled patient, although this latter possibility still remains speculative.

Coordination

While the studies discussed in the previous section treated gross motor responses, it is reasonable to expect that with technical variations even finer and coordinated movements can be conditioned, and there have been such efforts.

Minke and Heard (1964) worked with a five-year-old boy who had lost the coordination of limb movements on the left side of his body as the result of cardiac arrest occurring during surgery. Occupational therapists had been treating his left arm for three months with no effect, and his physician believed that he had no proprioceptive feedback from that extremity.

A translucent, plexiglass screen was mounted in front of the child. A slide projector could project eighteen circles of light onto the screen, the circles ranging in size from 18 inches to 1 inch in diameter. A red light was mounted above the screen, and a buzzer was located on the side. Foam rubber padding on the table in front of the screen protected the child's elbow.

There were three buttons for use by the experimenter. One of them turned the light on, one simultaneously turned the light off and sounded the buzzer, and one only turned the light off. A tape recorder presented white noise to the child, through earphones, for the duration of the light.

Reinforcement consisted of social interaction, occasionally followed by the delivery of a toy or a trinket. When a correct response was made, the buzzer sounded and the experimenter interacted with the boy by praising him and telling him that he liked him, or commenting on a remark which the child had made previously. Toys and trinkets were delivered on a VR5 schedule of reinforcement.

The child was seated in a chair which had a foot panel. Each of his legs was fastened to the chair with a strap. A strap was fastened about his waist and the back of the chair, and his right arm was strapped to his waist. The only movements he could make readily were bending his body above the waist, moving his head, and moving his left arm, which remained free. The strapping was imposed gradually, and the leg straps were removed during the negative reinforcement condition of the study.

The first phase of the investigation consisted of shaping the response of striking, with the left hand, an 18-inch circle of light projected on the plexiglass screen. The experimenter told the child to "hit the target" with his left hand. By the third session, shaping by successive approximations was begun, using social interaction as the reinforcer. The child was reinforced only if he responded when the red light was on; when the buzzer sounded, the light shut off and reinforcement was given. By the sixth session, verbal instructions were reintroduced as part of the general reinforcement, and in the seventh session the verbal prompt was faded out. By the ninth session, the response was developed sufficiently to proceed to the second phase of the study.

In this phase, the pretreatment condition, the child was reinforced for every arm thrust which resulted in his hand touching the screen, regardless of whether or not it struck within the projected circle of light.

The third phase involved selective reinforcement of responses which occurred within the area of the circle. Responses which were made outside of the circle of light resulted in the cessation of the red light, but the buzzer did not sound nor did the investigator interact with the child. If the child made eight or more correct responses within any ten trials with a particular circle, the circle was reduced in size by one inch. When he made two or less correct responses within any ten trials, the circle was increased one inch in size.

In the twenty-first session, a negative reinforcement contingency was introduced. The onset of the light was accompanied by noise presented through earphones worn by the boy. The termination of the light and of the noise were contingent upon the boy placing his hand inside the projected circle on the screen. This procedure was conducted in blocks of ten trials, and the circle was reduced in size following that block of trials in which twenty or less thrusts were made by the child. Any block in which fifty or more thrusts of the left arm occurred produced an increase in the diameter of the circle. Reinforcement was the same as during the other phases of the study.

In the twenty-third session, the response was redefined as having the fingers within the circle, regardless of the location of the hand which first touched the screen.

There were twenty-nine sessions of treatment conducted. The sessions were of twenty minutes duration.

The responses of the child to each circle are represented in Figure 4-3. The trials are grouped into blocks of ten each. The smallest circle, which could be presented to the child according to the general shaping criteria of the experiment, was 11 inches in diameter until the critical response was redefined. From that point on, progress proceeded rapidly and the child responded well, to even the smallest of the projected circles of light.

A technique employed by Minke and Heard which is not observed very frequently was termed "handicapping the handi-

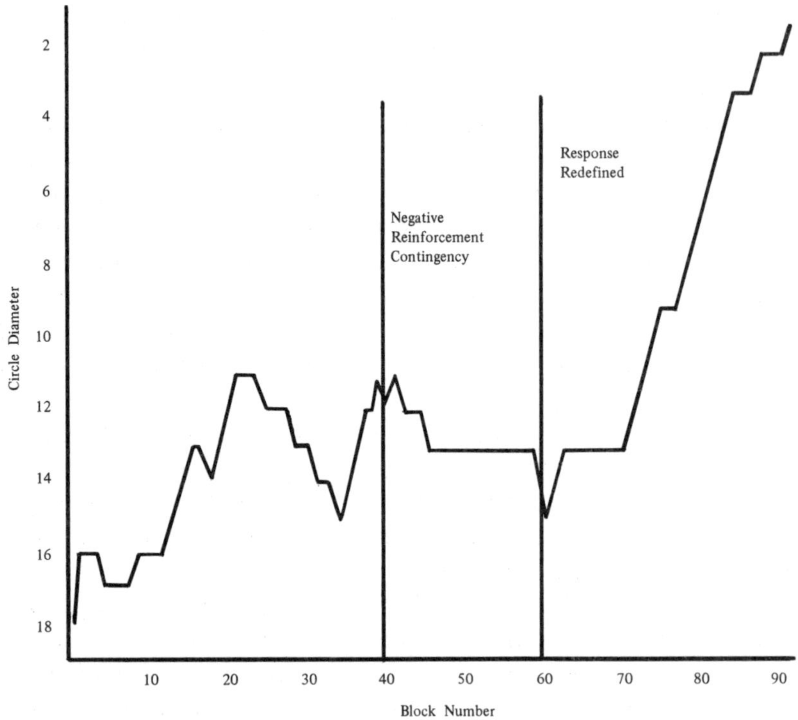

Figure 4-3 Responses of the child to each circle. Trials are grouped into blocks of ten. From Minke, K. A. and Heard, W. G.: The development of hand-eye coordination in a brain damaged child. Paper presented at the Annual Meeting of the Southwestern and Rocky Mountain Division of the American Association for the Advancement of Science, Lubbock, 1964.

Reproduced with the permission of the senior author and the American Association for the Advancement of Science.

capped," or restricting possibilities for responding when working with the physically disabled. This can be a very fruitful approach when treating a behavior for which an incompatible response has previously been reinforced. In the case of the child in the study, all of his manual movements had been made with the right, noninvolved hand. In the experiment right hand and arm movements were very strong, and even when reinforcement was contingent upon left arm movements, right arm movements generally preceded the reinforcer, and thus strength was maintained. Only when his right arm was immobilized by being strapped down did his left arm come to be used increasingly often, thus receiving reinforcement and being maintained. At the same time, his right arm was being reinforced for not moving, thereby at least partially extinguishing that behavior in the situation.

Occupational therapists and physical therapists are aware of substitute motions employed by patients with weakened muscles and they do try to control these. Perhaps, by handicapping the handicapped, a disabled patient can be improved as previously unused muscles and joints are made to respond, and reinforcement is directed toward these and withdrawn from other responses.

The investigators stated that a next step to be taken with the child they treated would be the shaping of tracking responses, a more complex behavior.

* * * * *

Sachs and Mayhall (1972) studied the effects of reinforcement on the tracking behavior of a brain-damaged adult. Their subject was an eighteen-year-old woman diagnosed as a cerebral palsied, tension athetoid quadriplegic. She had involuntary movement of all extremities, which was more pronounced in the arms and on the left side. In addition, the patient displayed intermittent rigidity of all extremities, which also was more severe on the left side. As a consequence of her disability, she had great difficulty holding a pencil and forming letters, turning the pages of a book, and dressing. Her intelligence, as measured by the Verbal section of the Wechsler Adult Intelligence Scale, was normal.

The behavior investigated was pursuit rotor performance. An electronic pursuit rotor, operated at a speed of 30 r.p.m., was connected to two electric timers used to time rotor trials and intertrial intervals. A timer clock wired into the system recorded the number of seconds during each one-minute trial that the subject remained on target. Auditory feedback was provided to the subject by an audio oscillator which generated pure tones of 700 hertz (Hz) or 1000 Hz at 60 db. An aversive stimulus, in the form of a buzzer, had an intensity of 78 db. All auditory stimuli were presented through a speaker. With the exception of the speaker, all apparatus were located in a room adjoining the experimental area.

The study was comprised of a series of procedures which were as follows:

1. *Baseline* — no contingencies were imposed for target tracking.
2. *Reinforcement and Tone Feedback* — three levels of positive reinforcement were employed.
   a. R+1 — Reinforcement consisted of two cents for every second on target within a trial, above the mean on-target performance for the three previous sessions. When the criterion was reached, the subject received a 1000 Hz tone to indicate that reinforcement was being earned.
   b. R+2 — This procedure was the same as R+1 for the initial five trials of a session. During the last five trials, reinforcement was raised to four cents.
   c. R+3 — Five cents were earned for every second on target over forty seconds. Tone feedback was given throughout the session for all on-target responses. A 700 Hz tone was employed until the forty-second criterion was met, and then the tone changed to a 1000 Hz tone to indicate the earning of reinforcement.
3. *Tone Feedback* — There were two levels of tone employed.
   a. Tone Feedback 1: A 1000 Hz tone was contingent upon on-target behavior when performance exceeded the mean on-target behavior of the previous three sessions.
   b. Tone Feedback 2: A 700 Hz tone was contingent upon on-target behavior throughout each trial.
4. *Non-Contingent Tone* — A 1000 Hz tone was presented randomly during each trial.
5. *Escape from Buzzer* — When the subject's response went off target, the buzzer sounded and remained on for the duration of off-target behavior.
6. *Escape from Tone* — A 700 Hz tone was presented, contingent upon off-target behavior, and remained on until the subject returned to target.

Figure 4-4 presents the mean time on target (TOT) for each

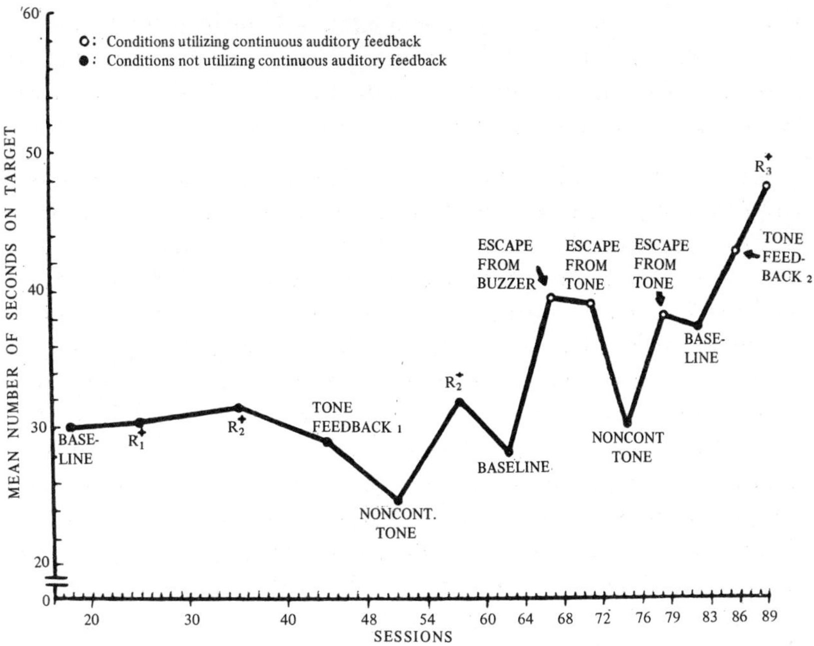

Figure 4-4 Mean number of seconds on-target (TOT) per condition. Each point represents the rate averaged over all trials and sessions within a condition. From Sachs, D. A. and Mayhall, B.: The effects of reinforcement contingencies upon pursuit rotor performance by a cerebral-palsied adult. *J Nerv Ment Dis, 155*:36, 1972.

Reproduced with the permission of the senior author and the *Journal of Nervous and Mental Disease*. Copyright 1972, the Williams and Wilkins Co., Baltimore, Maryland.

experimental condition. When reinforcement was contingent upon behavior which exceeded the mean behavior of previous sessions, as in R+1, R+2, and Tone Feedback 1, there was very slight improvement in TOT, and even a decrease in the last-named condition. During the conditions of *Escape from Buzzer, Escape from Tone,* Tone Feedback 2, and R+3, when the subject was reinforced for remaining on target, there was a highly significant increase in TOT. These conditions produced mean increases of 9.5, 9.1, 12.9 and 17.1 seconds respectively, from baseline performance. When the response contingency was removed, and

Non-Contingent Tone employed, responding returned to baseline level. Reinstatement of *Escape from Tone* resulted in a return to a higher level of performance. This demonstrated that improved performance was not a practice effect, but was a direct consequence of reinforcement.

Since Sachs and Mayhall treated a fairly complex behavior involving not only movement but coordination as well, the question may be raised regarding the practical and long lasting benefits which might be generated from a study of this nature. The authors feel that it might be possible, over many sessions involving external feedback followed by sessions during which this external cueing is faded, to effect permanent improvement in the control of movement by patients with cerebral palsy. In considering such a possibility, factors of age, extent and severity of disability, length of time since onset of disability, function of sensory systems, and motivation have to be taken into account. There is also the matter of generalization from the specific behavior which has been conditioned to other behaviors, and this can only be determined empirically.

Coordinated Movement Plus Function

Hesse and Friedlander (1974) believe that one of the reasons retarded, physically disabled children do not appear to have potential for effective motor ability is that they lack the appropriate opportunities to develop the skills of which they might be capable. By providing these opportunities in a structured and orderly manner, habilitation and rehabilitation programs for these children can prove beneficial.

The psychologists employed the PLAYTEST system with a seventeen-year-old boy with left-sided, spastic cerebral palsy. He also had a hearing loss, no speech, and a receptive language impairment. Furthermore, the boy was mentally retarded. The investigators dealt with the problem of minimal utilization of the left arm. Although the functional potential of this arm was restricted by the cerebral palsy involvement, it was felt that if the boy could develop the residual potential of the extremity, his proficiency in everyday tasks and his workshop performance would be enhanced significantly.

Two PLAYTEST consoles were used with this patient. The first consisted of a sequence of tasks which required him to turn a doorknob, operate a light switch, operate a screen door type of handle, and pull a drawer handle. These task modules were activated in random sequence by the control system every ten seconds.

The second console was comprised of six identical modules. Each one was a disc of red plastic five cm in diameter, mounted on a white, plexiglass panel, 12 cm X 20 cm. The modules were spaced at a distance of 18 inches between centers. The patient had to press the appropriate disc, as indicated by a cue light, with a force of 0.5 N, using a pointer which was 46 cm in length. The modules were activated in random sequence at a rate of every twenty seconds.

The training sessions were conducted four times per week for a total of five weeks. During the first two weeks the patient was permitted to perform the tasks with his right hand, but then was restricted to using only his left hand for the remainder of the experiment.

An independent measure was obtained of the patient's ability and his willingness to use his left hand, both before and after training.

A third console, which was similar in principle to the other two, required coordinated use of both hands for successful performance of the tasks it presented. The patient was tested with this during three sessions prior to, and three sessions immediately following the left-handed training sessions.

The reinforcement consisted of immediate auditory and/or visual feedback, such as music, flashing colored lights, and similar stimuli.

During the first two weeks of right-handed activity, the patient's performance was high and consistent. His time-on-task (the percentage of the session that he actually was touching one of the discs with the pointer), and correct response duration (the percentage of his total response time during which he was touching the correct disc with the pointer), exceeded 90 per cent. When he was required to use only his left hand, performance declined to 25 per cent, but from then on he made steady gains.

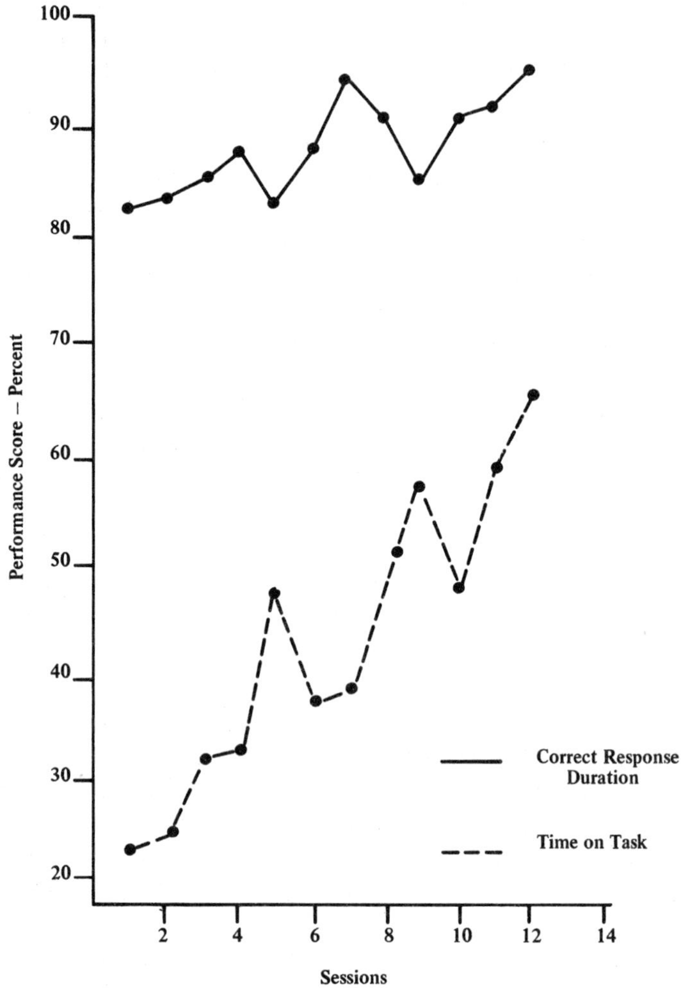

Figure 4-5 Record of left hand tool performance on an automated motor tracking task by a seventeen-year-old male with severe left side spastic cerebral palsy. From Hesse, G. W. and Friedlander, B. Z.: Behavioral training of a retarded adolescent to develop voluntary use of a previously unused CP involved arm and hand. (Unpublished manuscript)

Reproduced with the permission of the senior author.

The data for his left-handed performance are presented in Figure 4-5. Shown are his percentage time-on-task and his percentage correct response duration. As can be seen, his time-on-task score was initially low, and it improved progressively. His correct response score, which began high, also showed steady but less dramatic improvement. Increases in both scores, between the first three sessions and the last three, were significant. There was, therefore, true improvement in the patient's proficiency, and not merely an increase in speed at the sacrifice of accuracy or the reverse. There also was a significant gain on the pre- and post-training test which required coordinated use of both hands.

Soon after the training program had been initiated, the patient began to show increased reliance on his left hand to assist him in performing a variety of activities of daily living. This persisted, and the patient continued to use his left hand for many daily and manipulative activities such as holding and carrying objects; tasks which were not confined to those identical with the training tasks.

This study illustrates that, as mentioned previously when discussing the PLAYTEST system, not only evaluations but actual therapy can be conducted with this type of automated, operant-based apparatus. Hesse and Friedlander's results, and those of Friedlander et al. (1969) are all the more dramatic for the fact that they were obtained with patients who were not only extensively physically disabled but mentally retarded as well, often severely. They raise the possibility that no patient, no matter how impaired he may be, should be excluded from treatment, since with the appropriate procedures significant gains may be achieved even with those individuals who initially appear to possess very limited potential for improvement.

Finger Control

While arm movement and eye-hand coordination are necessary for upper extremity functioning, they are not always sufficient. If a patient is to utilize his movements functionally in day-to-day living, he must be able to use his hand. Movement of the hand and fingers in a utilitarian manner is extremely complex, and a study of it generally cannot be approached in a gross, molar way. The behavior must be broken down into its components, and these must be dealt with individually until a *gestalt* is achieved.

In a beginning effort, Sachs, Martin and Fitch (1972) improved motoric control of the fingers of an eleven-year-old girl with athetotic cerebral palsy. She displayed involuntary movements and incoordination of her head, neck, facial muscles and all extremities, and had great difficulty performing fine arm, hand and finger movements. In addition, she was functionally deaf and probably intellectually retarded. The patient's eight-year-old sister, who had normal motor development, served as a control subject in the study.

Five metal steel guitar picks were fitted onto the patient's fingertips. Each pick was covered with insulating tape, leaving only a contact surface of approximately 1 cm in diameter on the palmar side bare. Each pick was wired individually to the programming apparatus. Individual latencies were timed electronically. The timers could only be activated by sequential touches, i.e. from first finger through fourth finger or the reverse, depending upon the experimental condition.

Four amber lights, 1 cm in diameter each, were mounted in a row at 2.5 cm apart, on the diagonal surface of a box which measured 18 X 18 X 18 cm. A red light, 1 cm in diameter, was centered 4.5 cm below the amber lights. This was used to signal the start of a trial. The amber lights were activated in sequence to provide feedback to the patient when a correct touch had been made. Each amber light remained on until the next correct touch was made. All programming apparatus was located in an adjoining room out of the subject's sight.

The experimental procedure involved a left-hand digital exercise (LD), and a right-hand digital exercise (RD), as a control behavior. Each trial consisted of four finger-to-thumb touches, performed in sequence, from the fourth finger to the first for LD, and in the reverse order for RD. The control task required the use of the contralateral hand and the opposite order of responding so as to minimize bilateral transfer.

The critical response was defined as any completed touch in the proper sequence. Each session consisted oftwenty trials for each exercise. Whether LD or RD began a session was determined randomly. A two-minute rest period followed every ten trials to minimize fatigue. The experimenter entered the treatment room during the rest intervals to verbally encourage and praise the patient, thereby maintaining her motivation.

The experimental procedure was as follows: The patient was seated at a table with the light box on it. Her mother or father sat in a chair facing her, being instructed not to indicate approval or disapproval of performance by facial expressions or gestures. The picks were fitted onto the patient's fingers and the wires leading from the picks were taped to her forearm. The required behavior for the patient to imitate was demonstrated once. (During the first few sessions only, some manipulation of the patient's fingers was necessary for correct imitation.) Upon a signal, the parent instructed the patient to "get ready" for the red light which indicated the start of a trial. When the light came on, she was instructed to "go," but only if her palm and fingers were above the table and flat, and if she was looking at the light panel. Upon the completion of each trial the parent told her to "stop."

The patient was seen for a number of sessions, under different conditions, until stability had been achieved. Stability was defined as having been reached when, in comparing the last six sessions in a given condition, the difference between the mean of the first three sessions and the mean of the last three sessions was less than 15 percent of the mean of all six sessions. In conditions when six sessions could not be conducted, the criteria for stability were scaled down appropriately.

An equal number of sessions was conducted for LD and RD, with no experimental manipulations of RD. The experimental conditions for LD are listed below.

1. *Baseline* (B) — The patient performed the task with no lights or contingency conditions present.
2. *Non-Contingent Visual Feedback* (NVF) — The four amber lights came on in sequential order at random intervals. Activation of the lights was not contingent upon correct responding.
3. *Contingent Visual Feedback* (CVF) — The amber lights were lighted sequentially, contingent upon correct responses, i.e. touches. As each light came on, the previously

lit one shut off.

The study required three months to complete, and consisted of a total of thirty-six sessions. Between two and five sessions were conducted per week, no more than one session being held per day, with the exception of the last two days, when the patient had to return to school.

The control subject was treated in the same manner as the patient, but for fewer sessions. She wore padded earphones during the experiment so as to equate her hearing with that of the patient as nearly as possible.

* * * * *

The results of this investigation revealed that contingent feedback significantly improved responses beyond what might be expected as a result of practice alone.

Figure 4-6 presents the average total latency for the patient for both the LD and RD conditions. During the initial baseline period, her mean latency of responding for the LD task was 17.7 seconds, while for the RD task it was 17.9 seconds. NVF did not significantly reduce the latency for either activity. The CVF decreased the latency for LD to 5.2 seconds. The RD exercise, which did not have an external contingency, had a mean latency of 10.8 seconds. Reversal procedures, indicated by B_2 in the figure, increased the average latency of LD to 8.2 seconds. The mean latency for RD during this period was 8.0 seconds. When the contingency was reinstated, the LD latency was 4.7 seconds, and the latency for RD was 7.0 seconds. During the CVF condition, LD was superior to RD in 100 out of 120 trials.

The control subject showed no statistically significant difference between LD and RD for any of the conditions.

The individual latencies for each of the four touches for the LD exercise were reduced also for the patient under conditions of CVF. No such relationship was observed for the control subject.

An interesting possibility arising from a consideration of the procedures and results of this investigation is that feedback alone, and not necessarily feedback as a reinforcer, may be sufficient to modify responding. The authors are aware of this and point to the need for further research.

The importance of the study lies in the fact that a patient with

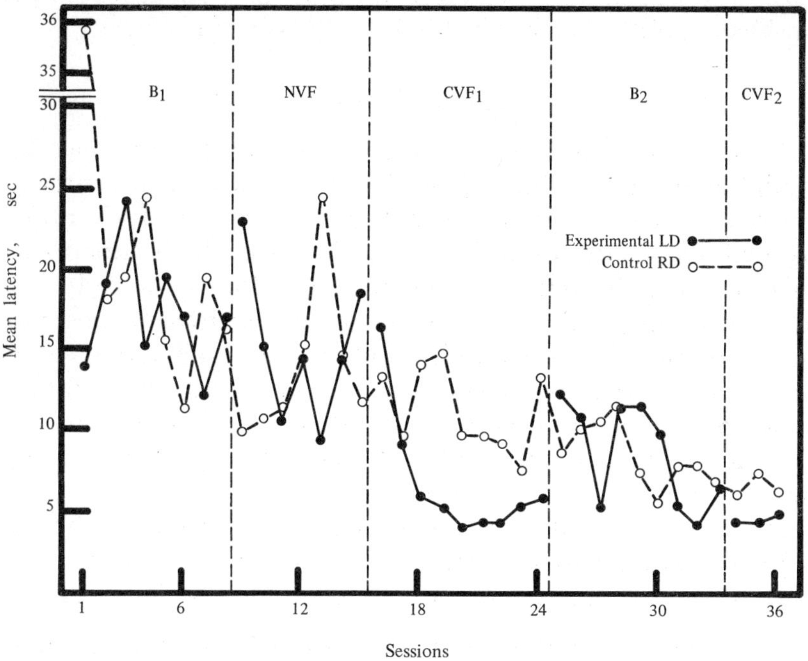

Figure 4-6 Mean total latency per session for LD and RD for *S*. The conditions, applicable only to LD, include baseline (B_1 and $_2$), noncontingent visual feedback (NVF), and a contingent visual feedback (CVF_1 and $_2$). From Sachs, D. A., Martin, J. E. and Fitch, J. L.: The effect of visual feedback on a digital exercise in a functionally deaf cerebral palsied child. *J Behav Ther Exp Psychiat, 3*:217, 1972.

Reproduced with the permission of the senior author and the *Journal of Behavior Therapy and Experimental Psychiatry*. Copyright 1972, Pergamon Press.

involuntary, uncontrolled movements of all extremities, who previously had difficulty executing fine upper extremity movements, was conditioned to make fine finger responses in a reliable and controlled way. This holds promise for training of disabled patients, and the possible extension of such training into daily living activities may be considered feasible. The cerebral palsied comprise a relatively large percentage of a rehabilitation patient population, particularly in institutions which have services for children. Not only might these children benefit from similar procedures, but adults with Parkinson's disease, multiple sclerosis, or any disorder in which involuntary movement presents a problem could also conceivably be helped in this manner.

Orthotic Training

An orthosis is a device which pertains to or promotes the straightening of a deformed or distorted body part. It assists or corrects a nonfunctioning, or malfunctioning part (Ince, 1974). An orthotic device, from the point of view of the occupational therapist, usually implies some type of splint or brace for an upper extremity. Splints vary not only with regard to purpose but in the complexity of their design and structure, and in the type of power supply required to operate them. Orthoses are important adjuncts to rehabilitation therapy and, for many patients with a permanent disability, they are indispensable for self-sufficiency in numerous areas of functioning.

Despite their utility, orthotic devices often are rejected by patients who, for a variety of reasons, prefer to be dependent rather than wear an orthosis which makes them more independent.

Trombly (1966) applied reinforcement techniques in training quadriplegic patients to use an orthosis.

The basic unit was a flexor hinge hand splint which fit over the patient's index, middle fingers, and thumb, and extended over the wrist and two-thirds of the forearm to provide stability. It was hinged at the metacarpophalangeal joints. When power was applied, the fingers were brought towards the thumb in palmar prehension. The fingers were pulled back into extension by a spring when power was released. With this device, the patient had to learn to control the degree of opening and closing so that objects ranging from a delicate potato chip to a 1-pound lead weight could be picked up without fumbling. The control device was placed at a site on the side of the body contralateral to the splinted side, a site where the patient could control muscle contraction and had sensation, and did not limit motion nor become active during the patient's usual motions. A ball bearing, forearm orthosis supported the patient's arm and permitted movement within a limited range through use of the noninvolved muscles and gravity.

The training which was conducted with one power source, an electric torque motor, will be described here. This motor drives a transfer cable which attaches to the splint and closes or opens the fingers by tightening or slackening. It is controlled by a clapper-type, three-position switch which drives the motor forward or in reverse, or holds it without action. In order to operate this power source, the patient must learn to: 1) push the clapper of the switch to its highest position, thus closing the fingers; 2) quickly release the switch to hold that position; 3) push the clapper halfway up, until he sees his fingers begin to open; and 4) "feather" the switch to close or open it in minute increments to pick up any particular object.

Initially, the patient was taught about the apparatus. The control was explained and demonstrated. Then it was put on him and he was given the opportunity to use it exploratorily. The therapist reinforced all correct movements by verbally praising the patient. She gave him a series of commands, involving the proper use of the device, and praised every correct response.

At first, any use of the control switch which was even nearly acceptable received reinforcement. Then, by successive approximations, the patient was shaped in his responding to make a sure closing of the splint, differentiating this from trial-and-error closings. Finally, only correct responses were reinforced and incorrect responses were extinguished through lack of reinforcement. Each drill period consisted of a series of grasp-and-release tasks with various objects, and at the end of the period the patient's score was compared with the score of his previous performance on the same tasks. When his performance exceeded past performance the therapist delivered reinforcement.

The first patient with whom this method was employed had been fitted with the unit three years prior to the study but gradually had refused to wear it unless the occupational therapist and his physician were present and insisted upon it. Follow-up of this patient after the termination of the reinforcement procedure confirmed that he was using the splint every day.

The second patient, who previously had required weeks of training to use a different device, learned to use the new unit satisfactorily within one week of training and continued using it correctly.

Trombly presents a possible explanation for the resistance of many patients toward wearing an orthotic device. She notes that the less a patient tries to become independent, the more attention he receives from the therapist. As he attempts to gain independence, the therapist tends to withdraw and leave him "on his own." When he is dependent, therefore, the therapist pays more attention to him in her efforts to encourage him to become independent than she does when he strives for independence. The therapist thus is reinforcing behavior in reverse of what the goals actually are. While a patient is refusing to wear an orthosis he receives positive reinforcement in the form of attention from the therapist as she tries to convince him to wear it. However, when a patient begins to use the device, the therapist feels able to turn her attention to other tasks while he practices alone. This withdrawal of reinforcement for desired behavior has the effect of extinguishing it. In her study, Trombly reversed the contingencies and achieved the desired results.

ADVANCED BEHAVIORS

Once the necessary and sufficient movements of the arm, hand and fingers have been achieved, the patient can progress to more difficult behaviors which are more closely related to his functioning as a member of society. Restoration of movement is only part of the total rehabilitation of a patient. For rehabilitation to be complete, the patient must be able to functionally utilize what he has gained in therapy.

There are also a number of patients who do not achieve return in their affected extremities. Most notable among these are patients with spinal cord injuries, and patients who have suffered a cerebrovascular accident and do not regain use of the involved arm and/or hand. These people must learn to use their unaffected extremity to perform the activities which they previously had done with the plegic limb or with both limbs.

Additionally, some patients, who have marked impairment of both upper extremities which cannot be corrected in a fundamental way, must come to use what they do possess in a functional manner within the limitations imposed by the disability.

The following studies provide examples of how some of these problems have been dealt with, and how further gains can be achieved in the disabled through conditioning techniques.

Typing

Ince (1973) improved the typing skills of a forty-year-old man who had suffered a stroke approximately nine months prior to the training. The CVA had resulted in a right hemiplegia with mild-moderate expressive aphasia, and a mild receptive aphasia. In his former profession, the patient had depended upon typing a great deal, an activity which his disability now made nearly impossible.

The patient was given the task of typing one line at a time from a standard typing exercise book in which all lines were of equal length. He had to perform this with his left hand because of the paralysis of his right upper extremity. His rate per line was timed with a stopwatch and recorded.

Following a baseline period of five 1-line trials, the patient was shown his scores (rate of typing per line), and was instructed to improve his speed. Verbal reinforcement, such as, "That's better," "Now you're doing well," and "That was very good," was given for each block of five 1-line trials in which there was a mean decrease in time per typed line from the mean of the previous block of trials. Upon completion of each block of trials the patient was shown his times, which provided him with further feedback regarding his performance. There were no other contingencies. Each session consisted of two blocks of trials. Since the patient's errors were minimal, they were not treated.

The results are depicted in Figure 4-7. Block 1 represents the baseline period, during which the patient averaged 119 seconds per typed line. Following this initial free operant period responding was variable, but by the fifth session the patient was typing at a markedly faster rate. His behavior began to indicate stability by the final four sessions. His rate of typing for the last block of trials was seventy seconds per line, a significant improvement over his baseline performance.

* * * * *

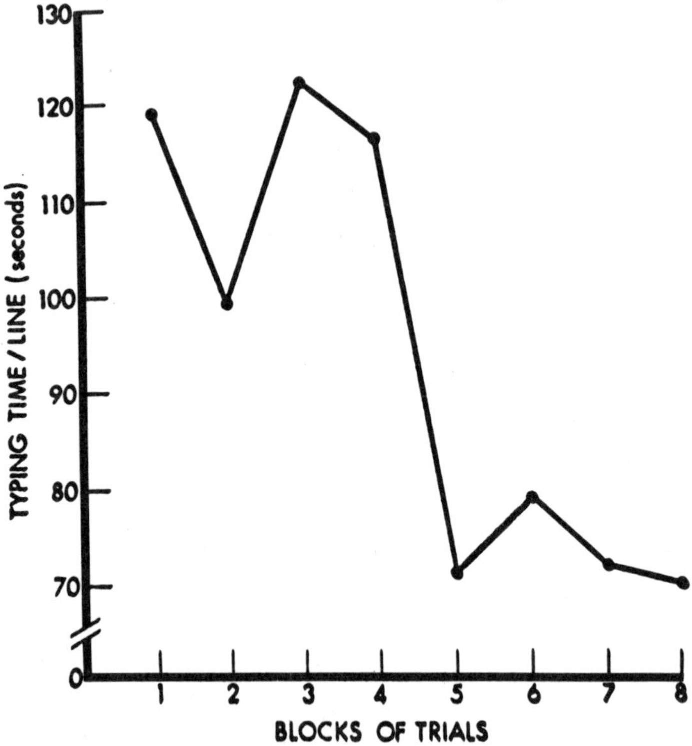

Figure 4-7 Mean rate of typing per block of trials. From Ince, L. P.: Behavior modification with an aphasic man. *Rehab Res Pract Rev*, 5:37, 1973.

Reproduced with the permission of the *Rehabilitation Research and Practice Review*, Arkansas Rehabilitation Research and Training Center.

Typing also was greatly improved by Ince (1968) in an eighteen-year-old girl with dystonia musculorum deformans. She had been coming to the hospital on an out-patient basis three times per week for three months, spending one hour each time in the prevocational shop of the Occupational Therapy Service.

As a consequence of severe muscular contractions, she was

using only the index finger of her right hand to type approximately twelve letters. This was followed by a rest period. Before she was able to resume her typing, she performed a wide, distorted, sweeping motion of her right arm, which she claimed relaxed her. During the entire time, her left arm was held rigidly, straight out behind her.

A combination of instructions and verbal reinforcement was employed to improve the patient's typing behavior. She was told how to sit at the typing table, where to place her hands, and how to move her hands back and forth from the table to the keyboard of the typewriter. When she followed these instruction correctly she was reinforced with, "That's right," or "That's better," or a similar praise statement. When she failed to respond correctly, no reinforcement was given.

The patient's behavior gradually was shaped by successive approximations beginning with reinforcement of any movement of her left hand towards the keyboard, and progressing until she was using her left hand to position the carriage. The shaping procedure was continued until she eventually was using all of the fingers of her left hand for keys on the left side of the keyboard, and the fingers of her right hand for the keys on the right side of the keyboard. Within a fairly brief period of time, both hands were being used appropriately.

The patient additionally was conditioned to type more words each time without a resting pause by verbally reinforcing improved production. This procedure was continued in her home. Her mother was instructed to have the patient type at least fifty words without a rest, verbally reinforcing correct movements and, upon completion of the task, to play one of the patient's favorite phonograph records. This latter step had the dual effect of reinforcing desired behavior and providing a short rest period.

Within two months, the patient's typing speed had increased from a baseline rate of approximately thirty words per hour to more than 120 words per hour. Whereas she formerly had to rest after typing only twelve letters, she now was able to type over sixty words without a pause. Furthermore, her grotesque motions were eliminated and she sat in a normal typing position using both hands properly.

It should be added here that following the progress made with typing, the same kinds of procedures were employed with ambulation and eating behaviors. In the former activity, she was instructed as to how to stand, how to point her feet, etc., and was reinforced verbally for ambulating increasingly longer distances without resting. Regarding the latter, she was trained and then reinforced for correctly holding utensils, and was shaped in eating behavior through reinforcement of accuracy in cutting and raising utensils to her mouth.

With these procedures she began by walking short distances such as 50 feet, and within a brief time was able to ambulate 150 feet without fatiguing as she formerly had. Her gait also became more normal in appearance. In fact, a staff member who had observed her ambulation was later questioned as to her opinion of the girl's performance. Her reply was, "I didn't know there was anything wrong with her."

The patient became able to use a knife and fork successfully with the modelling clay on which training was conducted, but remained fearful of using a knife at home with meat. However, she did use a fork at home and began feeding herself for the first time in years.

As a result of gains made in these areas, the patient was given instruction in self-dressing. With the psychologist guiding the occupational therapist regarding procedure, the patient rapidly learned to dress herself using buttons, zippers and snaps, a behavior she had not previously performed.

Contact with the girl's mother several months later revealed that she was about to enroll in college, an endeavor which had never been considered before.

Key-Punch Operation and Handwriting

A forty-one-year-old former key-punch operator had suffered a stroke following cardiac surgery. The CVA produced a right hemiplegia and moderate aphasia, both expressive and receptive. Approximately one year after the CVA she was placed on an occupational therapy program to relearn the operation of a key-punch machine. The work entailed correctly punching holes in IBM cards by means of an electronic keyboard. The patient previously had used both hands for this job, but now had to perform the work with her left, nondominant hand alone. After having performed this task daily for several months, she had made little progress in terms of speed of copying numbers, which she did very slowly.

At this point, Goodkin (1966) began to work with the patient. He recorded the length of time she required to punch each series of numbers on the IBM cards assigned to her, and computed the mean time per card per day for the activity. She then was given ten trials per day, in sessions which ranged from fifteen to thirty minutes in duration.

During the first two days, a baseline measure of the patient's performance was obtained. She averaged 110.6 seconds per card for this period.

The training consisted of telling the patient that she was doing well for improved times (verbal reinforcement), telling her how long it took her to complete a card (informational feedback) and, when she performed the task faster, informing her of how many seconds she cut off her previous best time (reinforcing feedback). When the patient responded more slowly than her previous time, she merely was instructed to go on to the next card. At the conclusion of each session the patient was informed of her mean time per card for that day, and this was compared with her performance on previous days.

Figure 4-8 reveals that within ten days the patient significantly reduced the length of time it took her to punch a card. Her performance is somewhat variable, but shows signs of stability over the last several days. While prior to the contingency procedures her time per card was more than 110 seconds, by the ninth day of training it was only seventy-one seconds.

Four months after completion of this study, the patient's occupational therapist informed Goodkin that, although the patient had been practicing handwriting with her left hand for more than one year, little progress had been made in speed of writing. The patient was frustrated and discouraged by this.

This problem was approached by recording the patient's per-

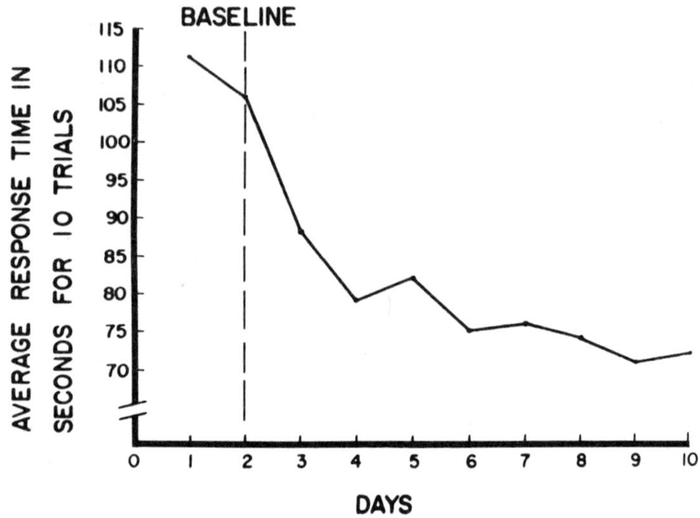

Figure 4-8 Changes in average response time on a keypunching task. From Goodkin, R.: Case studies in behavioral research in rehabilitation. *Percept Mot Skills, 23*:171, 1966.

Reproduced with the permission of the author and *Perceptual and Motor Skills.*

formance and reinforcing only faster writing. Periodic suggestions were made with regard to improvement, in an effort to correct errors more rapidly than by shaping alone. These consisted of suggesting the use of an underliner, encouraging the patient to look at two or three words before copying them, and to say two or three words aloud before writing them.

Initially, the number of letters copied from a paragraph during one-minute trials was recorded. The patient was given ten trials each session, with a thirty-second rest period between trials. At the end of each session, the mean number of letters copied per trial was calculated.

The first two sessions constituted a baseline period, and training began with the third session. The same basic procedure was applied to this problem as had previously been employed to improve the patient's key-punch operation. She was told that she was doing well (verbal reinforcement), was told the number of

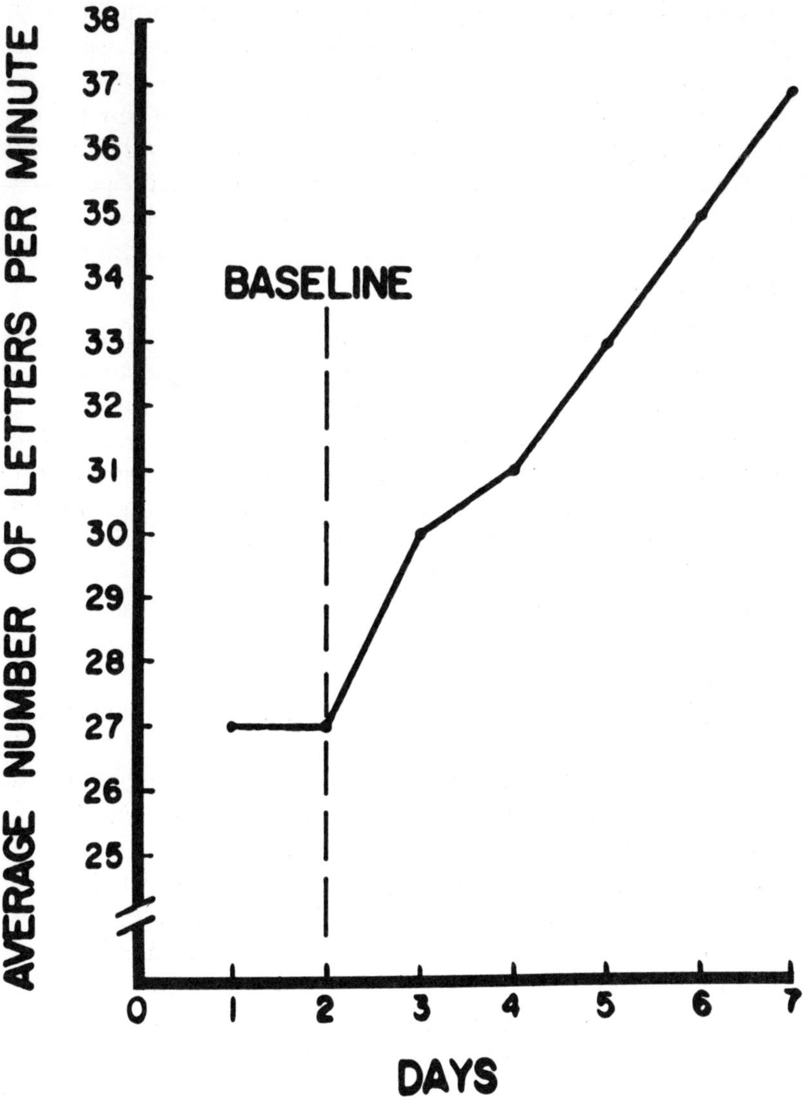

Figure 4-9 Changes in number of words copied per minute. From Goodkin, R.: Case studies in behavioral research in rehabilitation. *Percept Mot Skills, 23*:171, 1966.

Reproduced with the permission of the author and *Perceptual and Motor Skills.*

letters which she copied during the one-minute trials (informational feedback), and was told how many letters she added to her previous best score (reinforcing feedback). When she copied fewer letters than before she was told nothing.

The results are presented in Figure 4-9. It is clear that from the first treatment day the patient steadily increased in her speed of writing. The mean rate of copying during the baseline period was twenty-seven letters per minute. After only five days of behavior modification, she was copying thirty-seven letters in the same period of time.

The above studies illustrate several points. *First,* lost abilities can be restored or compensated for by appropriate behavior modification techniques. Loss of the use of one extremity does not necessarily mean total loss of function. Previously performed activities can be performed again by the disabled person through utilization of remaining abilities. Conditioning, and other behavior modification techniques, when properly applied, can accomplish much towards this end.

Secondly, not only gross motor behaviors, but those involving fine movements and skills can be trained, even in hands and fingers which previously did not perform such activities.

Third, the extent of a patient's disability should not necessarily be considered a variable in planning a behavior modification program. The eighteen-year-old girl who was helped by Ince was severely disabled in all extremities, and in her trunk and neck as well, yet a great deal was accomplished.

Fourth, a significant advantage of behavior modification is its systematized approach. Goodkin had observed that prior to his modification of key-punch performance, the patient had verbally been reinforced by her thearpist, but that this reinforcement was not being given contingent upon improved performance. Rather, it was delivered intermittently on a subjective basis. By carefully measuring performance on the task, he was able to deliver reinforcement systematically on the basis of objective data, and this is what produced the desired improvement.

REFERENCES

Block, J. D., Forster, S., Ma, P., Wietfeldt, Barbara and Murase, K.: Hemiplegic hand spasticity: Amelioration by assisted-extension practice with augmented feedback. Paper presented at the Annual Convention of the American Congress of Rehabilitation Medicine, San Juan, 1971.

Friedlander, B. Z., Gencheff, T., Moore, Marie and Nelson, Kay: Automated exercise procedures in evaluation and rehabilitation of upper extremity motor skills with seriously disabled institutional retardates. Paper presented at the Annual Convention of the American Association on Mental Deficiency, San Francisco, 1969.

Fuller, P. R.: Operant conditioning of a vegetative human organism. *Am J Psychol, 62*:587, 1949.

Goodkin, R.: Case studies in behavioral research in rehabilitation. *Percept Mot Skills, 23*:171, 1966.

Halberstam, J. L., Zaretsky, H. H., Brucker, B. S. and Guttman, Andrea: Avoidance conditioning of motor responses in elderly brain-damaged patients. *Arch Phys Med Rehabil, 52*:318, 1971.

Hesse, G. W. and Friedlander, B. Z.: Behavioral training of a retarded adolescent to develop voluntary use of a previously unused CP involved arm and hand. (Unpublished manuscript, 1974)

Ince, L. P.: Escape and avoidance conditioning of responses in the plegic arm of stroke patients: A preliminary study. *Psychon Sci, 16*:49, 1969.

Ince, L. P.: Behavior modification with an aphasic man. *Rehab Res Pract Rev, 4*:37, 1973.

Ince, L. P.: *The Rehabilitation Medicine Services.* Springfield, Thomas, 1974.

Minke, K. A. and Heard, W. G.: The development of hand-eye coordination in a brain damaged child. Paper presented at the Annual Meeting of the Southwestern and Rocky Mountain Division of the American Association for the Advancement of Science, Lubbock, 1964.

Rice, H. K., McDaniel, Martha W. and Denney, Sarah L.: Operant conditioning techniques for use in the physical rehabilitation of the multiply handicapped retarded patient. *J Am Phys Ther Assoc, 48*:342, 1968.

Sachs, D. A., Martin, J. E. and Fitch, J. L.: The effect of visual feedback on a digital exercise in a functionally deaf cerebral palsied child. *J Beh Ther Exp Psychiat, 3*:217, 1972.

Sachs, D. A. and Mayhall, B.: Behavioral control of spasms using aversive conditioning with a cerebral palsied adult. *J Nerv Ment Dis, 152*:362, 1971.

Sachs, D. A. and Mayhall, B.: The effects of reinforcement contingencies upon pursuit rotor performance by a cerebral-palsied adult. *J Nerv Ment Dis, 155*:36, 1972.

Trombly, Catherine A.: Principles of operant conditioning: Related to orthotic training of quadriplegic patients. *Am J Occup Ther, 20*:217, 1966.

SECTION III

BEHAVIORAL TECHNIQUES WITH DISORDERS OF COMMUNICATION

INTRODUCTION

IF ONE WERE TO select classes of behaviors by which to differentiate humans from organisms which are ranked lower on the phylogenetic scale, those involving the use of language would have to be considered as primary. While it may be true that animals communicate in various vocal and nonvocal ways, it is the use of symbolic language which is unique to humans and which has enabled mankind to achieve what it has. It is speech and language which make us "human."

Therefore, when an individual loses all, or part of his language abilities he is restricted seriously in his functioning, particularly in his interactions with others. Gestures and facial expressions, of course, are communicative, and along with language help us to express ourselves to our fellows. While these modes are utilized by language-impaired persons to compensate partially for their losses, they cannot fully replace verbal language.

The rehabilitation of communication disorders, thus, is crucial, and a great number and variety of techniques have been developed over the years to achieve this. This section focuses on behavioral methods which have been employed in treating disorders of communication.

Chapter Five

DISABILITIES OF SPEECH AND LANGUAGE

IN PROFESSIONAL USAGE, the term *speech* is used to mean the noncontent aspects of verbal behavior. These include rate, volume, rhythm, pitch, phonation, and the functions of the peripheral speech mechanisms. *Language* refers to the content variable of verbal communication, the verbal expression of ideas which permits functional communication between people (Ince, 1974).

SPEECH

Hypernasality

Roll (1973) treated two children whose speech intelligibility was impaired by hypernasality secondary to cleft palate. One patient was a ten-year-old boy with a unilateral cleft of the lip, hard palate and soft palate, all of which had been repaired surgically. The second subject of the study was a thirteen-year-old girl with a cleft of the soft palate. In addition to the nasal quality of all of her voiced sounds, she was unable to make plosive sounds without the emission of air through her nose.

Hypernasality was defined behaviorally as vibration of the walls of the nasal cavities during production of an English vowel or diphthong.

The subjects sat in a sound-treated chamber with a microphone placed approximately 6 inches in front of and 6 inches below the chin. The piezo-electric crystal from a Lafayette harmonica contact microphone was used to transduce the mechanical vibrations of the walls of the nasal cavities into electrical energy. The crystal was located on an adjustable rod which extended from a head band worn by the subjects.

At the start of each session, the crystal was placed firmly on the left side of the nose. The nasal passages remained open. The signals from the contact and acoustic transducers were amplified and relayed into a two-channel voice-operated relay system. A vocal response which did not produce nasal vibration activated a relay in the acoustic channel of the system, while a vocal response which did result in nasal vibration activated a second relay and prevented closure of the acoustic channel. The closure of each relay operated a separate counter.

In the feedback condition, when the relay in the nonnasal channel was closed, it resulted in the lighting of a 200-watt bulb located above the subject, markedly increasing the level of illumination in the chamber, which normally was lighted by a 60-watt bulb. When the nasal channel was closed, a 25-watt red light, mounted three feet in front of the subject at eye level, came on.

In order to insure the reliability of the measurement of the critical response, the dynamic microphone was calibrated to a preselected gain setting each day before the transducer was placed on the subject's nose. The subject then vocalized a sustained /m/ sound at an intensity which caused the Volume Unit (VU) meter to hover near zero, while the experimenter varied the position of the crystal until the voltage generated by the subject's nasal resonance was that recorded on the original crystal placement at the same vocal intensity. The voltage required to activate the nasal channel was set at 75 percent of the voltage generated by the /m/ utterance. The intensity of the vocal response necessary to activate the nonnasal channel was the same as that used for calibration. This prevented the subject from producing a false positive by speaking at a lower intensity. The calibrations were repeated at the conclusion of each session.

In order to select a response for modification, the subjects were asked in the first two sessions, via an intercom system, to repeat sounds made by the experimenter. He read a list of vowel and diphthong phonemes, repeating each sound randomly five times. The amount of voltage generated by the nasal transducer was recorded for each subject. The diphthong /eI/ as in the word "day," was selected as the response for the boy because it produced the smallest voltage change of all of the sounds which he consistently nasalized. For the girl, who nasalized all vowels and diphthongs at voltage levels near those produced by /m/, the /ɔ/, as in the word "all," was chosen because it was the vowel sound produced with the greatest opening of the mouth.

The sessions were conducted on a daily basis. The subject was seated in the chamber and the calibrations were performed. The child was asked to say either /eI/, or /ɔ/ until told by the experimenter to stop. There was a rest period of fifteen to twenty seconds duration following every ten repetitions. Each session consisted of 150 responses.

The experiment was composed of the following conditions:

1. *No Feedback*$_1$ — No feedback was given for any vocalization. The number of nasalized and nonnasalized responses was recorded. This condition was in effect until 250 responses had been made.
2. *Feedback*$_1$ — The subjects were given differential visual feedback for their responses. In the first session of this condition, each subject was told to continue repeating the defined response and that each correct vocalization would result in the white light coming on, while each incorrect sound would produce the red light. The lights were demonstrated manually to the subjects. They were instructed to try and make the white light come on each time they said the required sound.
3. *No Feedback*$_2$ — In this condition there was no feedback for correct or incorrect responding but the subjects were told to try and make the response which would turn on the white light.
4. *Feedback Reversal* — The instructions given to the subjects at the beginning of *Feedback*$_1$ were read to them again, but the light contingencies were reversed. Nasal sounds now resulted in the onset of the white light and nonnasal sounds produced the red light.
5. *No Feedback*$_3$ — Only the male subject received this condition, which was the same as *No Feedback*$_2$.
6. *Feedback Reinstated*$_3$— This condition was the same as *Feedback*$_2$. For the male subject it followed *No Feedback* , while for the female subject it followed *No Feedback* .

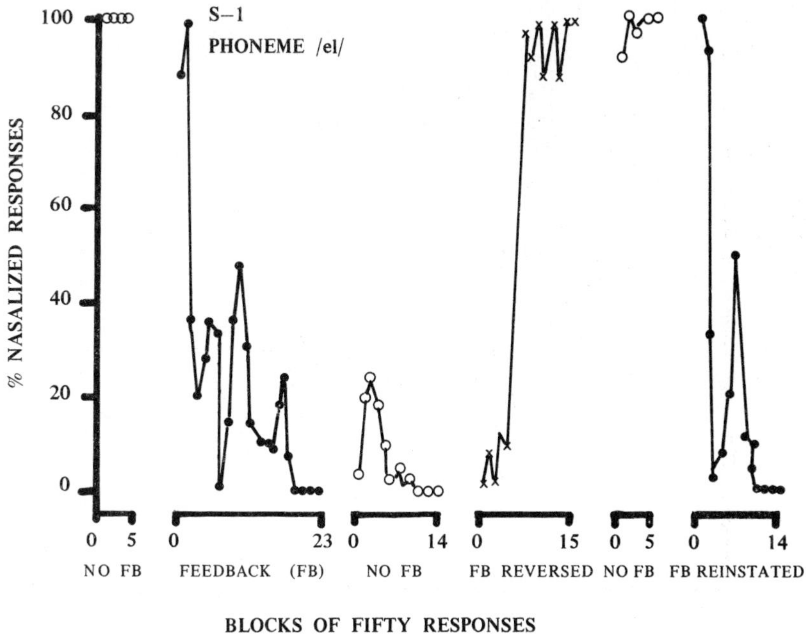

Figure 5-1 Percentage of /eI/ sounds nasalized by Subject 1 on each block of fifty trials under Feedback, No-Feedback and Reversed-Feedback conditions. From Roll, D. L.: Modification of nasal resonance in cleft-palate children by informative feedback. *J Appl Behav Anal, 6*:397, 1973.

The data for the male subject, Subject 1, are presented in Figure 5-1. When there was no feedback, all responses were nasalized, but differential feedback resulted in a rapid reduction of nasalized utterances. He met the criterion of 200 consecutive, nonnasal responses by the eighth session, and maintained good responding in the *No Feedback*$_2$ condition when he was requested to respond as if the lights were operative. When the light contingencies were reversed, the subject's responding also showed reversal. The *No Feedback*$_3$ condition resulted in the maintenance of the most recently correct response, with few errors. When feedback was reinstated, there was a rapid recovery of correct, nonnasal responding.

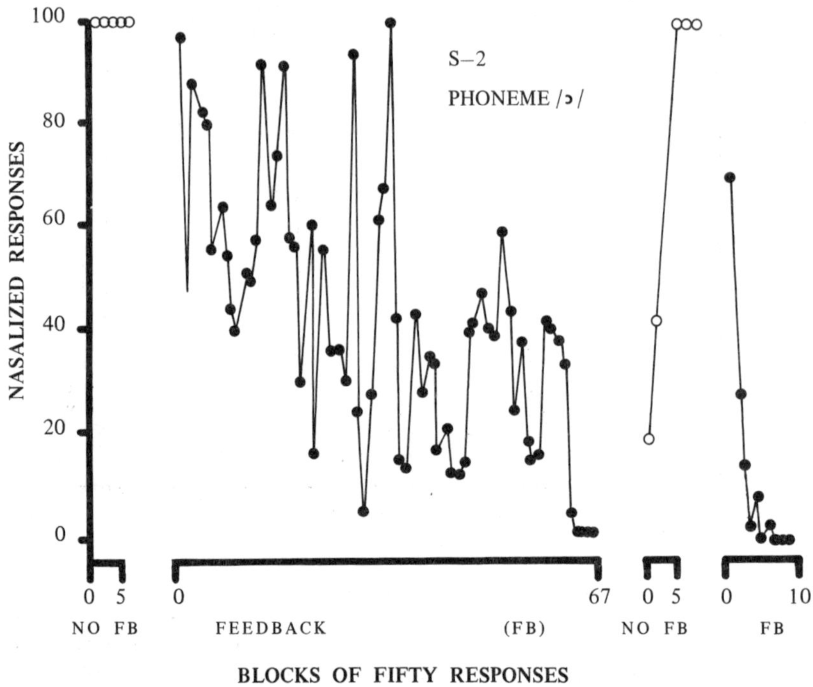

Figure 5-2 Percentage of /ɔ/ sounds nasalized by Subject 2 on each block of fifty trials under Feedback and No-Feedback conditions. From Roll, D. L.: Modification of nasal resonance in cleft-palate children by informative feedback. *J Appl Behav Anal, 6*:397, 1973.

Reproduced with the permission of the author and the *Journal of Applied Behavior Analysis*. Copyright 1973 by the Society for the Experimental Analysis of Behavior.

Figure 5-2 presents the results of the study for Subject 2, the female subject. When feedback was introduced it resulted in a slow trend towards nonnasalized speech until the criterion was met in the twenty-third session. Responding was variable, both within and between sessions. After much training the girl achieved good control over nasal resonance. In the first session of the *No Feedback* condition, the percentage of nasalized responses swiftly increased. When differential feedback was reinstated, nonnasal responding rapidly returned.

Differential feedback, therefore, was successful with both children in producing significant changes in the nasality of their speech.

While this study actually only demonstrated that control of the major place of resonance can be learned for an isolated vowel or diphthong, such techniques can be extended to more complex speech. A critical aspect of the investigation was the precision of the response definition. This is what gives the procedures certain advantages in speech therapy. In traditional speech therapy, a considerable time is often spent by the therapist describing to the patient how to use the palate to respond correctly. Roll had the subjects in his study spend the entire time emitting the critical response, deemphasizing instructions and providing contingent consequences for desired and undesired behavior. Specific requirements for speaking correctly were omitted. Thus, each subject could determine the most comfortable way of responding appropriately within his or her own physiological capability. Unless a response is adequately defined, it is very difficult to properly reinforce and measure desired behavior. In such a case, the results become uncertain, and the application of the methodology remains questionable.

Dysarthria

Dysarthria is one of the more frequently encountered speech disorders in rehabilitation, particularly among patients who have had a stroke, yet it is a problem which generally receives little attention in the literature.

Ince and Rosenberg (1973) extended the use of behavioral procedures to the modification of dysarthric speech in their treatment of two male patients.

One of the patients was a forty-nine-year-old man who had had a cerebrovascular accident approximately nine months prior to his participation in the study. He exhibited a moderate dysarthria characterized by impaired rate, articulation and voice quality. His articulation was marked by distorted sounds and errors of substitution and omission. He had a right-sided weakness of the oral peripheral speech mechanisms in a number of labial and lingual movements, and a severe impairment in rapid, repetetive articulation.

The other patient was fifty-two years-old. His CVA occurred seven months before the investigation began. He had a moderately severe dysarthria characterized by impaired rate, impaired articulation, low voice volume, and poor voice quality. He exhibited bilateral impairment of both labial and lingual movements, which were more pronounced on the left side. He also was deficient in diadochokinetic rate.

The functional intelligibility of both patients, as rated by their speech therapists, was poor. The prognosis for the first patient was considered to be fair, while for the second patient, it was felt to be poor/fair. Both men attended individual and group speech therapy daily, but progress was being made very slowly. The patients' speech therapists agreed to discontinue their therapy during the time behavioral procedures were applied to the problems.

Both patients were seen simultaneously by both experimenters for two thirty-minute sessions per week. They sat in their wheelchairs across a desk from the experimenters. A reel-to-reel tape recorder and microphone were located on the desk. A tape loop was employed instead of a standard reel, so as to permit immediate playback of recordings without the need for repeated rewinding of the tape and searching for the desired material. In front of the experimenters, on a board which was located below the level of the desk and unobservable to the patients, was a chart which was divided into two columns. One column was labelled *CLEAR,* and the other column was headed *UNCLEAR.*

The patients were instructed to speak in turn, on any topic they wished, and to speak only one sentence at a time. Thus, one patient spoke a sentence and both experimenters individually marked, with a "check," what they judged to be the appropriate column on the chart; then the tape was played back to the speaker. He was told whether or not his utterance was intelligible by one of the experimenters saying either "Clear," or "Unclear" to him, depending upon the judgements which had been made. When he was told "Unclear," the same experimenter repeated the sentence spoken by the patient, modelling it clearly and correctly. Then the patient had to repeat the sentence. Again, both experimenters made their notation on the chart. The tape was played back, and the patient was told "Clear" or "Unclear" by the second experimenter, who then modelled it correctly and intelligibly if it had been rated *UNCLEAR*. The patient had to repeat the sentence once more, and the experimenters marked the chart appropriately. The tape was played back, and both experimenters then said either "Clear" or "Unclear" to the speaker.

There were, therefore, three repetitions by the patient, three tape feedbacks, and three feedbacks from the experimenters, consisting of reinforcement for intelligible utterances, or punishment for unintelligible statements. When the procedure was completed with one of the patients, the other patient took his turn, and the entire procedure was repeated.

If the experimenters disagreed in their judgement of the intelligibility of a patient's verbalization (one experimenter marking the column labelled *CLEAR*, and the other marking the *UNCLEAR* column), the patient's utterance automatically was treated as if the judgement were one of *UNCLEAR*. When both experimenters agreed that a sentence had been spoken clearly, the tape was played back to the speaker and both of them reinforced him by saying "Clear." No further treatment was given for that sentence.

The study was terminated when the patients reached a criterion of three consecutive sessions without a single sentence rated as *UNCLEAR*.

Table 5-I illustrates the total number of recorded intelligible and unintelligible sentences spoken by both patients during the investigation. Approximately 15 sentences were verbalized by each patient per session. Thus, each block of sessions represents about 75 sentences for each patient. The last block represents only three sessions, or 45 sentences, because both patients reached criterion in this block.

It can be seen that initially Subject 1, the forty-nine-year-old man, had 67 sentences rated as *UNCLEAR*, and only nine rated

Sessions	Subject 1 Total number "unclear" sentences	Subject 1 Total number "clear" sentences	Subject 2 Total number "unclear" sentences	Subject 2 Total number "clear" sentences
1-5	67	9	72	4
6-10	57	18	69	6
11-15	39	35	49	25
16-20	30	46	33	43
21-25	18	59	20	57
26-30	7	68	8	67
31-35	2	73	3	72
36-38	0	45	0	45

Table 5-I Total number of recorded unintelligible and intelligible sentences per subject per block of experimental sessions. From Ince, L. P. and Rosenberg, D. N.: Modification of articulation in dysarthria. *Arch Phys Med Rehabil, 54*:233, 1973.

Reproduced with the permission of the *Archives of Physical Medicine and Rehabilitation.*

CLEAR, and that the fifty-two-year-old patient, Subject 2, had 72 sentences judged *UNCLEAR,* and only four which were determined to be *CLEAR.* However, from the initial five sessions, both patients steadily improved in the clarity of their speech, and during the final three sessions neither one uttered any unintelligible sentences. The major gains were achieved between the tenth and the fifteenth sessions for both patients, and also between the fifteenth and the twentieth sessions for Subject 2, but progress was regular and consistent throughout the study, with no reversals for either man.

Following the conclusion of the investigation, interviews were conducted by the experimenters with the patients' former speech therapists, nursing personnel of the patients' ward, rehabilitation therapists from other services, and other patients. All persons interviewed were unanimous in their views that both patients spoke much more clearly and now were completely intelligible.

Several techniques were employed by the psychologists, including positive reinforcement for correct responses and punishment for incorrect responses, immediate feedback of response for self-correction, modelling and practice. Which one of these, or which combination of techniques was most effective in achieving the results cannot be determined without replicating the study in a way that each variable is systematically controlled. Although such a determination is important from the standpoint of research, from a practical consideration it is sufficient to note that behavioral methods were successful in correcting the articulatory defects.

An interesting feature of this investigation is the use of two experimenters to treat two patients simultaneously. This was done to at least partially avoid the possibility of a single experimenter, in whose presence alone the patients would respond correctly, becoming a discriminative stimulus. Having more than two experimenters would have technically been unwieldy.

Vocal Quality

Not all speech impairments are caused by, or exacerbated by organic pathology. Some problems have a definite psychological component which can interfere with even the most intensive therapeutic efforts. This was the case with a sixty-four-year-old man treated by Ince (1968).

The patient had sustained a CVA with resultant mild aphasia approximately one month prior to being seen by Ince. The patient's speech therapist and psychologist had both observed that there were certain specific situations during which his speech became worse. That is, his voice developed a hoarse, strained quality, and his word-finding problem became more severe. Since his aphasia was quite mild, the determination was made to improve the vocal quality of his speech.

The patient was interviewed by the psychologist who learned that he was continually anxious regarding his former job. He had retired the previous year, but apparently was such a valued employee that his former employer still made entreaties to get him to return to work. The patient was chronically fearful that he would have to go back to work, which he did not want to do. However, he was the kind of individual who had always found it difficult to refuse requests, and felt that if pressure continued from his former superior he would yield. The situations in which he was asked to return to his job, as well as the anticipation of these situations, maintained his state of heightened anxiety.

Systematic desensitization was selected as the treatment of choice. A hierarchy of anxiety-provoking scenes was constructed by the patient and the psychologist. The scenes consisted of the following:

1. receiving a letter from a former co-worker requesting the patient to return to work;
2. receiving a telephone call from a former co-worker requesting him to return to work;
3. receiving a letter from his former employer requesting him to return to work;
4. receiving a telephone call from his former employer requesting him to return to work;
5. being visited in the hospital by his former employer who attempts to convince him to return to work.

Over a period of five 30-minute sessions, the patient was taught to relax through techniques described by Wolpe (1958). Then each scene of the hierarchy was presented to the patient by the psychologist, while the patient was deeply relaxed. He was requested to raise a finger each time he felt anxious while visualizing a scene. The scenes were presented one at a time, beginning with the first one on the list and proceeding until the fifth and final scene had been worked through without the patient indicating feelings of anxiety to the psychologist. There were three sessions conducted per week. Each session was approximately forty-five minutes in duration.

By the sixth desensitization session, the patient reported no longer feeling anxious upon being presented with any of the scenes listed in the hierarchy. He was able to visualize them clearly, and displayed no overt signs of nervousness. He stated that he no longer felt upset, tense, or bothered by them in any way. He also was able to speak freely about his former job and his desire to remain in retirement without the marked speech disability which formerly had accompanied such thoughts. On the weekend following termination of therapy he was, in fact, visited by his former employer and two former co-workers, and was able to remain calm and relaxed throughout their visit despite the conversation frequently pertaining to his old job. He reported that he had none of the hoarseness and straining of his voice which initially had prompted treatment.

Approximately two weeks after the termination of therapy, the patient contacted the psychologist and requested to be seen again. An interview with him disclosed that there were several hospital situations which made him anxious and resulted in the vocal impairments. Since systematic desensitization had previously been successful, it was employed again.

It required three sessions to relax the patient deeply, and under conditions of relaxation the following scenes were presented to him in hierarchical order, from first through fifth:

1. patients on his ward expressing to him that they thought he was either deaf or "stupid." (This was due to their lack of understanding his expressive aphasia.);
2. seeing other aphasic patients;
3. being ordered about by other patients during recreation activities;
4. being taken advantage of by other patients, i.e. being asked to do favors, having items borrowed, etc.;
5. patients and attendants "needling" him when he returned from weekend passes about always having to return to the hospital.

These scenes previously had been described and ranked by the patient. They were presented to him individually and, as before, the patient was instructed to raise a finger each time he experienced anxiety while visualizing a scene. Therapy was conducted five times per week, during forty-five minute sessions.

After three weeks of therapy, or fifteen desensitization sessions, the patient no longer indicated feeling anxious during the presentation of any of the hierarchy items. He was followed up via daily informal interviews for two weeks, and then in weekly interviews until his discharge from the hospital. Throughout this time period of several months, during which he repeatedly was confronted by all of the former anxiety-arousing situations, he evidenced no indications of anxiousness and reported feeling calm at all times. The hoarse, strained voice qualities which had once presented problems for him did not reoccur.

There are times when a patient's performance is affected adversely by fear or anxiety. This was seen in some of the studies reported in Chapter Three (Meyerson, Kerr and Michael, 1967; Di Scipio and Feldman, 1971) with regard to ambulation activities, and is true of verbal behavior as well, as the present investigation illustrates. Therefore, it benefits the members of the rehabilitation team to be alert to factors other than the physical disorder which may be handicapping a patient.

LANGUAGE

Evaluation of Comprehension

One of the basic problems in the area of language dysfunction is the determination of the receptive component of a patient's language loss. Many of the basic texts in the field either ignore the problem or devote little space to it, and in clinical practice the majority of therapeutic efforts usually are directed toward the improvement of expressive functions. Often it is assumed, as in the case of an aphasic patient for example, that the patient's inappropriate responses are almost entirely the result of an expressive language impairment, with little consideration given to the possibility that he may have a receptive problem which precludes correct expression. This is true particularly of young children who have difficulty conveying to the examiner or therapist the precise nature of the communication problem.

In an attempt to determine impairments of comprehension in children with language disabilities, Putzer and Friedlander (1970) tested preschool children's preferential selection between two sound tracks while the children watched television programs. One sound track presented normal sound, while the other presented sound which was so degraded by ascending levels of white noise interference that it became increasingly incomprehensible to adults with normal hearing. The investigators assumed that if a child failed to reject the degraded sound track it would mean that he had some primary disorganization of receptive language processes. This would imply that the child would not be able to understand what others said to him.

Three groups of preschool children were tested. One group consisted of language-impaired children without hearing loss, and the other two groups were comprised of normal children of the same age. One of these groups had a median range IQ, and the

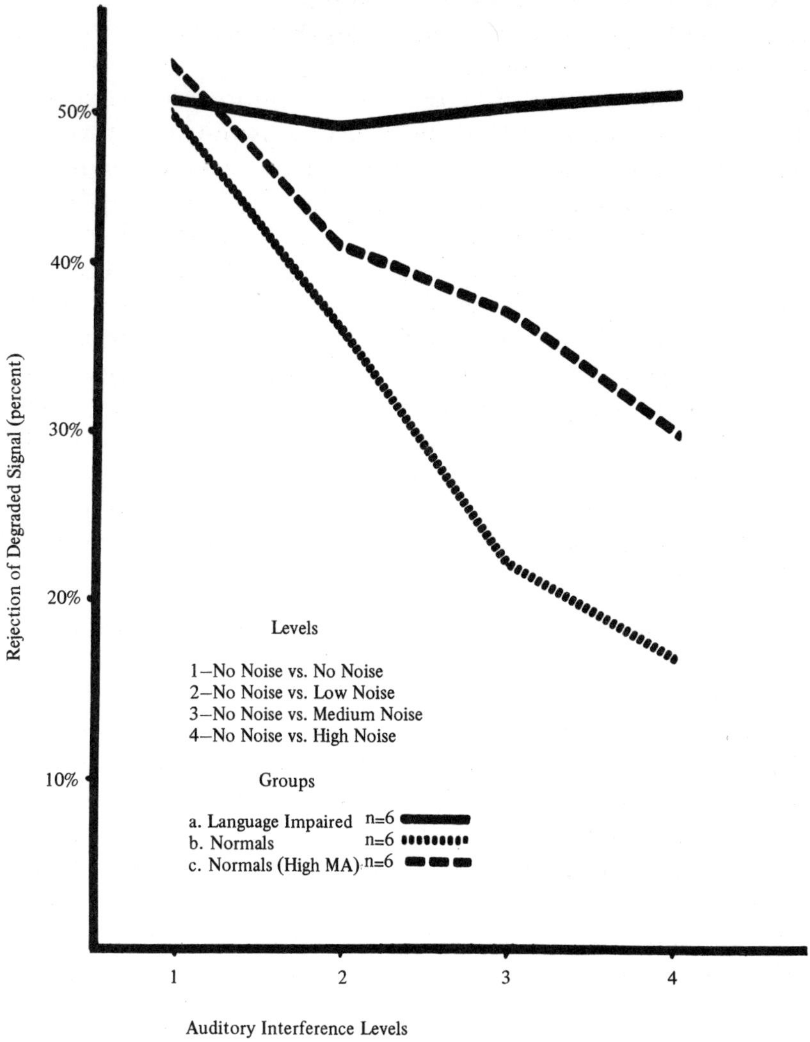

Figure 5-3 Effects of stimulus degradation on discriminative listening to television sound tracks by three groups of preschool children. From Putzer, R. K. and Friedlander, B. Z.: Effects of language status and audio stimulus degradation on preschool children's discriminative listening in an automated operant television game. Paper presented at the Annual Meeting of the American Speech and Hearing Association, New York, 1970.

Reproduced with the permission of the junior author and the American Speech and Hearing Association.

other group had an IQ in a high range.

The different degrees of sound track degradation were presented in separate sessions.

The results are seen in Figure 5-3. The figure reveals that while the normal-hearing children became increasingly rejecting of the degraded sound tracks as the noise interference increased in intensity, the language-impaired children did not. This group listened to the normal and the increasingly incomprehensible sound tracks with nearly identical degrees of attention. In addition, the auditorily-impaired children's listening response time was as high as that of the normal children. This means that the nondeaf children spent as much time listening, with the same high level of attention and interest, to television shows wherein the speakers were totally incomprehensible as to the same speakers when they were clear and easy to understand. This obviously indicated a disorder of language input recognition which made it impossible for them to differentiate between true speech and nonunderstandable auditory stimuli.

This study points out the importance of distinguishing between expressive and receptive components of language loss, and indicates that far greater understanding is required of the latter aspect, comprehension, than is known at present. It raises two legitimate questions: When a child exhibits a language loss or impairment, how much of what is perceived as an expressive disorder is actually the result of a receptive dysfunction?, and, How can a child be trained in therapy to express himself more correctly if he cannot understand what is being said to him, or does not receive correct exteroceptive feedback of his own speech? More studies of the type just described are obviously needed.

Aphasia

Aphasia probably is the most common deficit of language behavior observed among rehabilitation patients. This language loss or impairment, which is due to brain injury, may result from trauma or disease, but in a rehabilitation population it most frequently is associated with a cerebrovascular accident where the brain damage usually has occurred in the dominant hemisphere.

Within a brief period of time, Ince (1973) was able to improve the word-finding ability of an aphasic man. The patient was forty years old, and had suffered a stroke nine months prior to being seen experimentally. His language behavior was characterized by a mild-moderate expressive aphasia and a mild receptive aphasia.

The investigator observed the patient during several of his speech therapy sessions, and noted that the therapists were working towards improving the patient's phrase and sentence production. However, he had considerable difficulty with the expression of single words. He spoke with much hesitation, and with a long latency between a question and his response. It was decided, therefore, to attempt to improve his vocabulary of single words, the rationale being that if he were not fluent with single words he could not be expected to produce complete sentences.

The word category selected for improvement was nouns. The patient was seen for two 15-minute sessions per week. He was given the task of pointing to and naming objects in the experimental room, which was the investigator's office. His goal was to name as many objects as he could within a sixty-second time period.

Initially, a baseline measure of his ability to name objects was obtained during a block of five consecutive sixty-second periods or trials. During this period, no feedback of any kind was given to the patient for his performance. Following the baseline phase, the patient was informed of his scores, i.e. the number of objects named per trial, and the mean number of objects named for the five trials, and was instructed to improve his performance.

Verbal reinforcement then was given to the patient for each block of five sixty-second trials in which there was a mean improvement in the number of objects named over the previous block of trials. The reinforcement consisted of statements of praise, such as, "That was better," or "Now you're doing better," or "That was more than before," and the like. At the conclusion of each block of trials the patient was shown his scores regardless of whether or not he had improved over the previous block. When he did not improve he received no feedback from the experimenter other than being shown his scores. Each experimental session consisted of two blocks of trials.

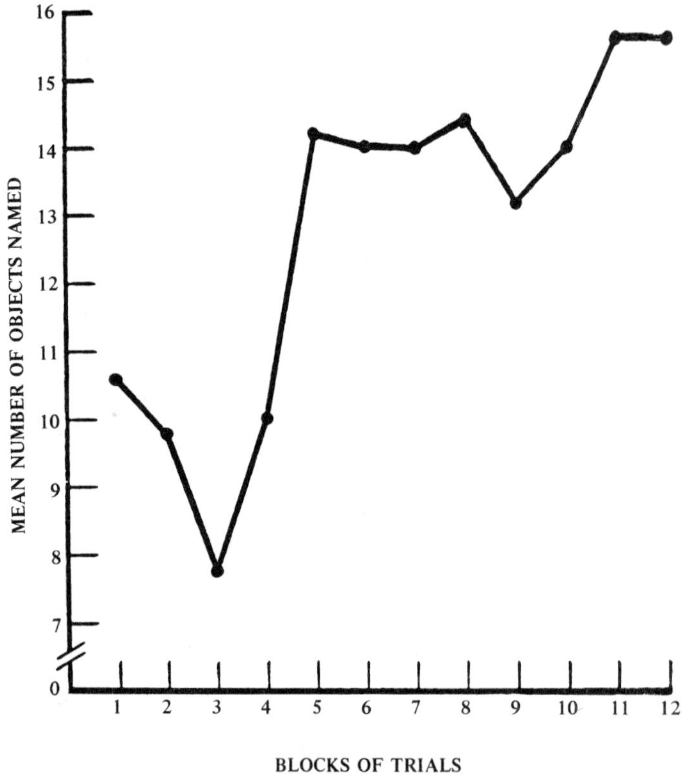

Figure 5-4 Mean number of objects named per block of trials. From Ince, L. P.: Behavior modification with an aphasic man. *Rehab Res Pract Rev,* 537, 1973. Reproduced with the permission of the *Rehabilitation Research and Practice Review,* Arkansas Rehabilitation Research and Training Center.

The data are presented in Figure 5-4. Within twelve blocks of five sixty-second trials, the patient's responses rose from a mean of 10.6 objects named per minute to a mean of 15.6. Block 1 represents the baseline period. The decline in responding seen to have occurred during the first two reinforcement sessions, Block 2 and Block 3, probably is attributable to the anxiety which the patient stated he felt in the novel situation. From the fourth block of trials, the patient's response rate rose with some variability. After the twelfth block of trials, the investigator left the hospital where the study was being conducted, but another psychologist continued the treatment in the same manner and reported further gains.

The fact that progress was made so swiftly in this case (a 50 percent improvement in responding within three weeks) probably is attributable to the decision to change the thearpeutic goal from phrase and sentence production to improved fluency with single words. Unless a patient has an adequate vocabulary which he can use readily, it is difficult for him to produce complete sentences. Learning single words appears to be a prerequisite for improved functional language of more complex verbalizations. Proceeding slowly in small steps can lead to greater and more rapid progress than an approach which attempts to accomplish too much too soon.

The feedback which the patient received concerning his scores also probably aided in his improvement since he was an intelligent, motivated individual who could make use of such information. The 1970 study by O'Brien and Azrin (see Chapter Three) previously had demonstrated that with motivated persons feedback of performance can result in improved behavior. While not all patients can benefit from informational feedback, withholding such data from those who can may retard progress.

It is interesting and important to note that when the original investigator left the institution, another psychologist was able to continue the work with the patient. This was possible because a basic feature of operant conditioning is its technological precision, even when not conducted in an experimental laboratory. Improved patient functioning should never be dependent upon therapist variables, only upon methodological ones. When procedures are specified clearly, it should be possible for almost anyone to be trained to carry them out with the desired results.

* * * * *

Some of the most important work in the operant treatment of aphasic patients has been conducted by Goodkin, and the remainder of this section is devoted to his investigations.

In 1966, Goodkin worked with a man who had had a CVA resulting in right hemiplegia and a moderate-severe expressive and receptive aphasia. The patient was making little progress in speech therapy, and perseverated a great deal in his verbal expressions, tending to repeat responses which were inappropriate to the stimuli presented to him. In addition, he exhibited little generalization of correct responding from one therapy session to the next.

The goals of the behavior modification program were determined to be an increase in the frequency of understandable words and phrases that the patient emitted in response to relatively unstructured questions, a decrease in the frequency of unintelligible responses, and a decrease in the frequency of perseverations.

Each day, the patient was orally presented with ten questions to which he had to respond for two minutes. The questions were as follows:

1. Tell me about this room. What are some of the things you see in the room?
2. Tell me about your clothes. Describe the clothes you are wearing.
3. Tell me about your classes here (in the hospital). What classes do you have and what are you doing in them?
4. What kinds of things do you do outside of your classes?
5. Tell me about where you live. Describe your home.
6. Tell me about your family. Tell me about some of the people in your family.
7. Name as many animals as you can.
8. Name as many cities and towns as you can.
9. Tell me a little about New York City.
10. Tell me a little about (name of the hospital).

Good responses were defined as utterances which included at least one clearly distinguishable word. Bad responses were those utterances that consisted of repeated words or indistinguishable sounds.

One session was conducted per day. The first five sessions constituted a baseline period. Beginning with the sixth session, responses to Questions 1, 4, 5, 7 and 9 were treated as follows: Good responses were reinforced by the experimenter giving the patient a verbal compliment, or commenting on their correctness and repeating the response, e.g. "That's right. It's a desk." Bad responses caused the experimenter to shake his head negatively, but not respond verbally. Questions 2, 3, 6, 8 and 10 were designated as noncontingent questions. The experimenter did not respond in any way to the patient's answers to these questions.

As evidenced in Figures 5-5 and 5-6, this treatment had little influence on the patient's performance while it was in effect from Days 6 through 13.

On Day 14, a new procedure was introduced. Each good response by the patient was followed by a compliment and a repetition of the response by the experimenter. Then he pointed to a box containing blue poker chips, from which the patient took one chip. If the patient's verbalization was a bad one, the experimenter informed the patient of the nature of his error, i.e. repetition or unintelligible utterance, and pointed to a box of red poker

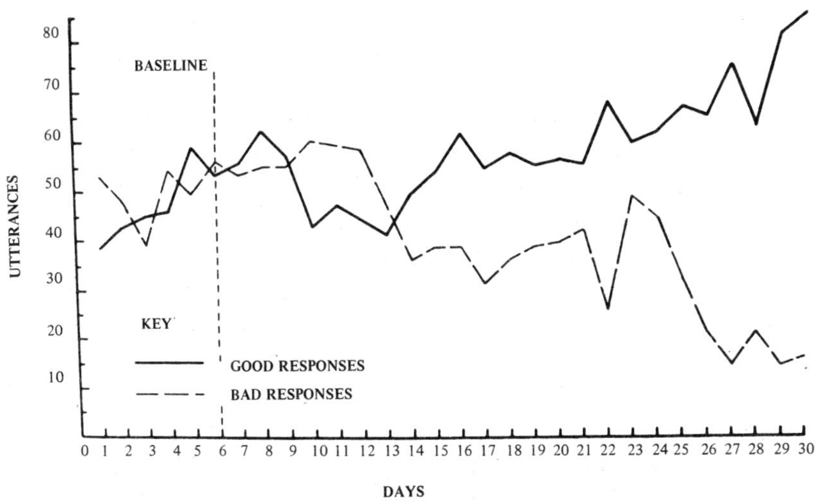

Figure 5-5 Total frequency of good and bad utterances per session. From Goodkin, R.: Case studies in behavioral research in rehabilitation. *Percept Mot Skills, 23*:171, 1966.

Reproduced with the permission of the author and *Perceptual and Motor Skills.*

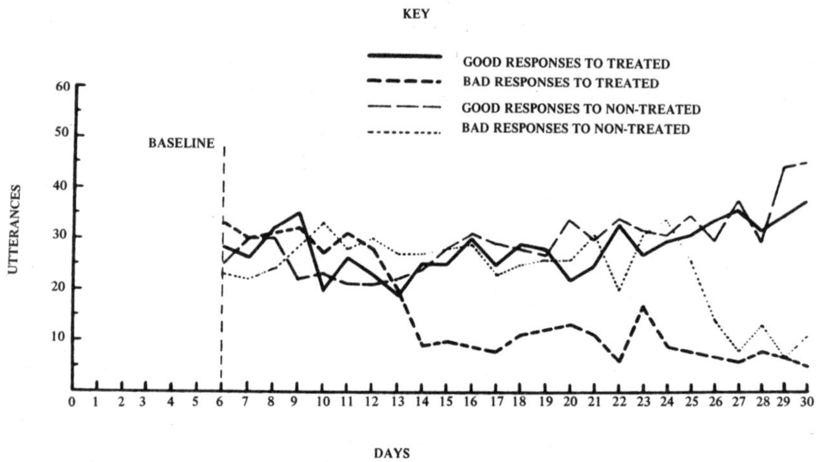

Figure 5-6 Good and bad utterances to treated and non-treated questions. From Goodkin, R.: Case studies in behavioral research in rehabilitation. *Percept Mot Skills, 23*:171, 1966.

Reproduced with the permission of the author and *Perceptual and Motor Skills.*

chips from which the patient took one chip. At the conclusion of each session, the experimenter added up the total of blue chips earned by the patient. As the figures show, this technique, which continued for seven sessions, markedly reduced the frequency of bad responses to the contingent questions.

On the twenty-second day, a modelling procedure was introduced. The experimenter responded to each of the questions for one minute. His responses included several good verbalizations, two repetitions, and one unintelligible utterance during each of five modelling periods. Following each good response, he reinforced himself with a compliment, a repetition of the response, and a blue poker chip. Following each bad response, he punished himself by naming the type of error he had committed, and taking a red poker chip. This technique, as seen in the figures, resulted in the most intelligible responding and the fewest errors committed by the patient up to that point.

The remainder of the study, Sessions 26-30, consisted of having the patient select a blue poker chip for every good response and a red chip for each bad response, without being told by the experimenter whether his responses were good or bad. During noncontingent questions, the boxes containing the poker chips were closed. The patient reinforced or punished his own responses during the two-minute response periods. Then the experimenter responded to the patient's verbalizations by reinforcing or punishing them with the appropriately colored chips. Each time a red chip was given, the patient was informed of the reason for it. At the conclusion of responding for each contingent question, the number of red and blue chips taken by the patient was compared openly with the number given by the experimenter.

This condition of the study resulted in a significant reduction of the patient's bad responses to noncontingent questions which, until this time, had been the same as the number of good responses to these questions. This effect is seen in Figure 5-6.

* * * * *

Goodkin (1966) employed a similar approach with a woman who had sustained a cerebrovascular accident with consequent aphasia of three years duration. She used many words, but tended to shift rapidly from one topic to another. Furthermore, her answers to questions generally were inappropriate.

The patient was presented with the same ten stimulus questions which had been employed with the previously discussed male patient, and she too had to respond to each question for two minutes. Verbal reinforcement and a blue poker chip were given, contingent upon each fifteen-second period during which her response contained material which was relevant to the question. After each fifteen-second period which did not include relevant material, she was informed of her error and given a red poker chip. In fewer than fifteen treatment sessions this patient exhibited a significant reduction of irrelevant responses to the stimulus questions.

Goodkin's initial study is interesting from the point of view of several procedures being employed with a single subject over a relatively brief period of time. He utilized verbal reinforcement, confirming repetition as feedback, gestural punishment, token reinforcement, informative feedback, token punishment, modelling, self-reinforcement, and self-punishment, all within twenty-five days following baseline measurements. This illustrates that in behavior modification there are times when the investigator must be flexible in his approach. Although it is desirable to predetermine the experimental procedures, it is foolhardy to continue them when the desired results are not forthcoming, or are being achieved too slowly for the purposes of the study. Furthermore, behavior modification procedures always are tailored to the needs of the particular individual being treated, and are never rigidly employed in a universal way.

Dividing the number of stimulus questions into the number of those which were treated and those which were not permitted the investigator to have an ongoing control condition. Thus, information was provided continuously regarding the effectiveness of the techniques.

The fact that each technique which was used was systematically applied and controlled made it possible to replicate features of the study with the second patient and achieve success in her case as well.

In a subsequent investigation, Goodkin (1969a) again used several behavioral techniques in dealing with a number of response dimensions of an aphasic patient.

The patient was a fifty-six-year-old man with both sensory and motor aphasia, secondary to a CVA which had occurred two years previous to being seen by the psychologist. He had considerable difficulty in articulation, and had a significant word-finding loss. His expressive abilities were more severely impaired than his receptive capacity.

The patient was treated three times per week, during sessions of approximately thirty minutes duration. A baseline of responding was obtained for each new response category prior to the initiation of a treatment procedure. In addition, the patient's responses in the categories being dealt with had to demonstrate stability over at least three sessions before a treatment technique was introduced. Stability was defined as a variance of not more than from five to ten responses.

During each session, the patient was required to respond for two minutes to one of four sets of ten questions. These were the same types of questions used by Goodkin in the 1966 studies. Each day, five questions were selected for treatment. The other five questions were untreated, and served as a control for determining generalization of responding from the treated questions. When an improvement in one dimension of responding had stabilized, new response categories were selected for treatment. The response categories were treated in the following order:

PHASE 1. Building Word Frequency

A. Frequency of words and phrases emitted

B. Frequency of unclear utterances and perseverations

PHASE 2. Building Relevancy

A. Frequency of relevant utterances

B. Utterances that were clear, but unrelated to the stimulus question

C. Unclear responses and perseverations

PHASE 3. Building Sentences

A. Frequency of sentences

B. Frequency of words and phrases not in sentences

C. Frequency of unclear responses and perseverations

The following were the definitions of the response categories:

Words and Phrases — Words or phrases emitted that were not in the context of a sentence;

Unclear — Utterances emitted that were not recognizable words;

Perseveration — Any words that were repeated which did not express new material in response to a question;

Relevant — Words and phrases emitted by the patient which did pertain specifically to the stimulus question;

Irrelevant — Words and phrases emitted by the patient which did not pertain specifically to the stimulus question;

Sentences — A group of words contining all of the grammatical elements of a sentence, even if errors were made in grammar, or if they contained perseverations;

The experimental procedures and their definitions were as follows:

B (Base rates): The number of responses emitted in a category during a two-minute response period without experimental manipulation;

VR (Verbal reinforcement): Responses by the experimenter, such as, "Correct," "Very good," "That's right," "Right, it's a desk," and the like, which conveyed to the patient that his response was in a category designated to be increased;

VP (Verbal punishment): Responses of the experimenter, such as, "I didn't understand that," "You have already said that," "That wasn't a sentence," etc., which conveyed to the patient that his response was in a category designated to be decreased;

TR (Token reinforcement): The delivery of blue poker chips for responses by the patient in a category which had been selected to be increased;

TP (Token punishment): Red poker chips were delivered to indicate to the patient that his response was one selected to be decreased;

STR (Self-token reinforcement): When the patient responded in a category designated to be increased, the experimenter pointed to a box of blue tokens and the patient took one and placed it on the table before him;

STP (Self-token punishment): When the patient's response was in a category selected for reduction, the experimenter pointed to a box containing red poker chips, from which the patient withdrew one and placed it on the table in front of him;

M (Modelling): The experimenter gave responses in both the category to be increased and the category to be decreased, and reinforced or punished himself verbally and with the appropriately-colored poker chip; the patient began his own two-minute response period following one minute of this modelling by the experimenter;

DF (Delayed feedback): After each response during the two-minute period, the patient reinforced or punished his own responses without any cues from the experimenter; following this the experimenter restated each of the patient's responses and either reinforced or punished them;

DVR (Delayed verbal reinforcement): The experimenter reinforced responding after the response period;

DVP (Delayed verbal punishment): The experimenter delivered punishment after the response period;

DTR (Delayed token reinforcement): The experimenter dis-

Phase 1 Building Word Frequency

Step	Sessions	Procedure	Treated			Non-Treated			Total		
			Words & Phrases	Uncl. & Persev.	Sum	Words & Phrases	Uncl. & Persev.	Sum	Words & Phrases	Uncl. & Persev.	Sum
1.	1-5	B–Series 1							46	48	94
2.	6-8	VR-VP	29	31	60	28	23	51	57	54	111
3.	9-11	VR-TR	35	32	67	22	23	45	57	55	112
4.	12-14	VR-STR	23	29	52	22	30	52	45	59	104
5.	15-17	VR-STR-VP-TP	19	20	39	22	27	49	41	47	88
6.	18-20	VR-STR-VP-STP	27	9	36	28	27	55	55	36	91
7.	21-23	VR-STR-VP-STP-QR	28	12	40	27	26	53	55	30	85
8.	24-26	M	30	11	41	32	28	60	62	39	101
9.	27-30	STR-STP-DVR-DTR-DVP-DTP	35	7	42	38	10	48	73	17	90
10.	31-37	B–Series 2							61	20	81
11.	38-40	M-STR-STP-DTR-DTP	26	10	36	30	6	36	56	16	72
12.	41-45	B–Series 3							75	12	87
13.	46-48	M-STR-STP-DTR-DTP	41	4	45	39	2	41	80	6	86
14.	49-55	M-VR-VP	57	4	61	45	3	48	102	7	109
15.	56-59	B–Series 4							92	15	107
16.	60-62	M-VR-VP	44	3	47	47	5	52	91	8	99

Phase 2–Building Relevancy

Step	Sessions	Procedure	Treated				Non-treated				Total			
			Relev. Wds. & Phrases	Irrelev. Wds. & Phrases	Uncl. & Persev.	Sum	Relev. Wds. & Phrases	Irrelev. Wds. & Phrases	Uncl. & Persev.	Sum	Relev. Wds. & Phrases	Irrelev. Wds. & Phrases	Uncl. & Persev.	Sum
17.	63-65	B–Series 1									93	25	18	136
18.	66-68	VR-VP	45	5	8	58	37	11	4	52	82	16	12	110
19.	69-71	M-VR-VP	49	4	11	64	43	7	3	53	92	11	14	117
20.	72-74	M-VR-TR-VP-TP	46	3	4	53	44	7	6	57	90	10	10	110
21.	75-79	VR-VP	45	1	4	50	45	8	5	58	90	9	9	108

Phase 3–Building Sentences

			Treated				Non-treated				Totals			
			Sent-ences	Wds. & Phrases	Uncl. & Persev.	Sum	Sent-ences	Wds. & Phrases	Uncl. & Persev.	Sum	Sent-ences	Wds. & Phrases	Uncl. & Persev.	Sum
22.	80-85	B–Series 3									33	73	21	127
23.	86-89	VR-VP-STR-STP	19	27	3	49	18	28	10	56	37	55	13	105
24.	90-92	M-VR-VP-STR-STP	17	28	1	46	15	33	11	59	32	61	12	105
25.	93-95	B–Series 1									51	51	16	118
26.	96-98	M-VR-VP	28	12	2	42	30	14	4	48	58	26	6	90

Table 5-II Procedures and average number of responses in several response categories made by an aphasic patient. From Goodkin, R.: Changes in word production, sentence production and relevance in an aphasic through verbal conditioning. *Behav Res Ther*, 7:93, 1969.

pensed blue poker chips after the response period;

DTP (Delayed token punishment): The experimenter dispensed red poker chips after the response period;

QR (Questions reversed): The five questions previously receiving treatment were not treated, and the five previously untreated questions received treatment.

Table 5-II presents the results of the study. Inspection of the table reveals that the mean baseline frequency of words emitted was forty-six, and that this increased to a mean of 102 during Sessions 49-55. The base rate of unclear utterances and perseverations was 48, and by Sessions 49-55 this had decreased to only seven. The frequency of clear but irrelevant utterances decreased to nine by Sessions 75-79 from an initial rate of 25 during Sessions 63-65, when this category initially was measured. During Sessions 80-85, 33 sentences, and 73 words and phrases not in sentences were emitted. By sessions 96-98, these figures had changed to 57 sentences, and 26 words and phrases not in sentences.

The most effective of the numerous procedures used were self-punishment (Sessions 18-20), modelling (Sessions 24-26), and delayed feedback (Sessions 27-30).

There also appeared to be generalization of the conditioned responding. Each new series of questions began with baseline response rates that reflected more appropriate responding than previous base rates. In addition, responses given by the patient to nontreated questions increasingly approached those given to the treated questions. Furthermore, tests administered to the patient by speech therapists, upon conclusion of the study, showed a marked improvement associated with the conditioning procedures. The patient's family and staff members of the hospital reported more effective communication by the patient.

Goodkin's determination of the order of treatment for the various response dimensions was based upon logical considerations and not on systematic programming research. He chose to rank the categories in the order of the difficulty which they presented for the patient. This was done because the desired goal was improved language ability for the individual. The investigator demonstrated that paying attention to the immediate needs of a patient does not mean abandoning sound scientific procedure.

* * * * *

Some of Goodkin's most important contributions have been in the area of training spouses to improve the language ability of aphasic patients (Goodkin, 1968, 1969b, 1970; Goodkin, Diller and Shah, 1972). One of his major studies (Goodkin et al., 1972) is examined here in detail as representative of this research.

Twenty-three aphasic patients and their spouses, or spouse-surrogates, served as the subjects. They were subdivided into an experimental group of seventeen aphasic-spouse pairs, and a control group of six such pairs. Most of the patients were seen after at least a two-year post-CVA interval. Reinforcement and other procedures were in effect on a response contingent-basis for the experimental group members, while the control group received these techniques on a random basis.

The general plan of the investigation consisted of the following:

A. Obtaining a full day's sample of verbal behavior between a husband and his spouse at home, both before and after experimental treatment. This was accomplished by having the patient wear a small, wireless transmitter in his shirt pocket. The transmitter recorded continuous talking for up to twelve hours at a time, and was triggered only when the patient or another person in the same room spoke. After a five-second silence period, it stopped recording automatically.

B. Obtaining samples of verbal behavior in a controlled environment. While observing the aphasic patient and his spouse through a one-way mirror from a room adjoining the experimental room, the investigator had the spouse ask the patient ten open-ended questions. The patient responded to each question for two minutes. (The questions were similar to those used by Goodkin in his earlier studies.) The patient's spouse wore a single earphone through which she alone could hear the investigator. All verbal interactions between the patient and his spouse were recorded.

C. Developing a system for analyzing the verbal behavior of both the patient and the spouse.

There were seven patient categories or target behaviors to be increased or decreased.

1. ***Sentence***— A group of words containing all of the grammatical elements of a sentence. Grammatical errors and per-

severations did not affect the scoring;

2. ***Words and Phrases*** — Words and phrases emitted which were not in the context of a sentence;
3. ***Unclear*** — Utterances not understood as recognizable words;
4. ***Dysfluency*** — Nonfluent speech, e.g. drawing out the beginning of a word as in "sssstore," or sounds occurring between words, such as "uhhh" or "err,"
5. ***Perseveration*** — Repetition of a word or words without expressing new content in response to a question. An example of this type of response is, "A desk over there" "A desk here," "A desk there," etc., in response to the question, "What are some of the things you see in this room?"
6. ***Direct Answer*** — Any word or words emitted which specifically relate to the question asked;
7. ***Self-Correction*** — A response in which the patient himself states that he made an error in what he said, or when he began his verbalization again and revised it.

There were eight spouse categories or target behaviors to be increased or decreased.

a. *Positive Feedback* — Words which conveyed the message that the patient's response was clear and correct, e.g., "That's right," "Mmmhmm," "Good," and the like;
b. *Objective Negative Feedback* — Feedback which was task-oriented, such as "I didn't understand that," or "You have said that already," or "That wasn't a sentence;"
c. *Subjective Negative Feedback* — Feedback that was person-oriented. For example, "Is that all you can say about it?" or "No good," or "You should do better;"
d. *Additional Questions* — Questions asked during the patient's two-minute response period after the initial stimulus question had been presented;
e. *Modelling* — Giving examples of appropriate answers to the stimulus questions;
f. *Starts Word* — Filling in the first letter or syllable of a word which a patient appeared to be trying to say, and permitting him time to say the entire word himself;
g. *Immediately Supplies Word* — Supplying a word which the patient appeared to be trying to say within five sec-

onds after the patient spoke his last word;

h. *Supplies Word After Waiting*—Supplying a word which the patient appeared to be searching for after waiting more than five seconds after the patient spoke his last word.

D. Obtaining measures of the spouses's personality which might affect her effectiveness as a trainer. Katz's adaptation of the Edwards Personal Preference Schedule (EPPS) was employed for this purpose. Nurturance was the main variable assessed.

E. Evaluating the effects of the techniques. The Functional Communication Profile (Taylor, 1964), which assesses the functional communication of aphasics, was administered to the patients by speech therapists prior to and following speech therapy, and following the experimental treatment. The spouses also completed this form prior to the study.

F. Teaching the spouses principles and techniques of behavior modification. Following the measurement of base rates of responding, each spouse was given a brief, individual course in the principles and methods of behavior modification. Techniques of shaping, reinforcement, punishment, extinction, modelling and fading were discussed and related to how the spouse was responding to the patient, and how these responses can be modified to bring about improved patient speech. Base rate tapes also were reviewed with the spouses in terms of which of the patients' target behaviors were to be increased, decreased and modified.

Then the spouse and the patient were observed by the experimenter from an adjoining room through a one-way mirror. The spouse asked the patient the various stimulus questions, and the experimenter gave her feedback and suggestions concerning her responding to the patient in view of the goals which had been set. Communication with the spouse was accomplished by means of the earphone which she wore during the sessions.*

There were several operant conditioning procedures employed in the experiment. They were selected on the basis of having been demonstrated as effective in previous research (see Goodkin, 1966, 1969a). The techniques were as follows:

---

*Baseline rates were defined as three consecutive sessions without a deviation in responding of more than five in any category for both the patient and the spouse. The baseline data were used to select the categories to be modified in the study.

1. Verbal reinforcement
2. Verbal punishment plus red tokens
3. Verbal reinforcement plus blue tokens
4. Modelling
5. Self-reinforcement
6. Self-punishment
7. Patient reinforces spouse. The spouse intentionally gave both appropriate and inappropriate responses, depending upon the patient's specific errors, and the patient verbally reinforced her behavior.

Each treatment was continued until the responses of each patient and spouse category had stabilized. The criterion for stability was the same as that used to determine the base rates.

After a minimum of fifteen sessions, new base rates were obtained, both in the patients' homes and in the experimental setting. Pre- and post-treatment Functional Communication Profiles were administered by speech therapists to the patients and their spouses, who also completed the Katz adaptation of the EPPS prior to the experimental sessions.

During the experiment, the topics to be discussed and the methods of eliciting verbal behavior from the patients were determined individually. The nature of the topics, the frequency of topic changes, and the treatment methods employed were dependent upon the level of each patient's functional speech and his interests. Patients who were at a low functional level received the same series of questions for many sessions, while for those patients with a higher level of language function, the topics were changed more often, and were selected from their known general and daily interests.

The spouse and the experimenter focused on each patient's specific deficit, e.g. increasing clear words, phrases and sentences, or decreasing unclear or perseverative utterances, and on the content of the patient's speech.

There were six individualized treatment procedures utilized, in addition to the general procedures described above.

1. An attempt was made to give each patient more awareness of the adequacy of his response. After each verbalization, the patient had to indicate if he felt his response was correct or not. The

spouse verbally reinforced or punished this self-judgement.

2. With patients who had difficulty in repeating specific sounds, the presented stimuli and the patients' voices were magnified through an amplifier and a set of headphones. The loudness cue gradually was faded until the headphones were no longer used.

3. Twelve patients had portions of the taped sessions with their spouses played back to them. This enabled them to hear themselves, and to hear the effects of their interactions with their spouses, who also listened to the playbacks. The experimenter commented on specific responses which they made while they listened to the tapes.

4. The experimenter substituted for the spouse with several of the patients to model correct procedures while the spouse observed the sessions through the one-way mirror.

5. Systematic desensitization was employed with three patients to reduce their level of anxiety.

6. Fading, or errorless learning, was used in two ways. With some of the patients who were at a low functional level of communication, the objects they named were visually introduced. Then the presentation of the visual cues were faded out and the patients had to name the items. In the second method, the patient's spouse modelled whole words for four or five sessions, with the patient repeating these words. Then, for the next four or five sessions, the spouse said only the sound of the first letter or syllable of the word, and the patient stated the entire word. Finally, the spouse only asked a general question concerning the practiced words, to which the patient had to respond without receiving any auditory cues.

This novel experimental study produced several significant results. The mean change for each experimental patient target behavior was 14.9 percent in the laboratory, while the control patients changed 4.4 percent in the opposite direction, i.e. negatively. In the home environment, the experimental patients exhibited a mean change of 12.5 percent, and the controls showed only a 5.4 percent change. The spouses in the experimental group had a mean target change of 11.6 percent in the laboratory, and 3.0

percent at home. The corresponding figures for the spouses in the control group were -3.0 percent and -2.3 percent, respectively.

The median verbal output per target category of the experimental patients increased from 80 to 114 responses in the experimental setting, and from 15 to 20 responses at home. The control patients increased from 35 responses at baseline to only 36 responses in the laboratory setting, and from 11.5 to 16.0 responses in the home environment. These verbal output scores refer to the total frequency of clear sentences, words, and phrases emitted by the patients during the response periods.

The Functional Communication Profile scores of the experimental group increased significantly as a result of the behavioral treatment, while those of the control patients did not increase.

The total mean percentage change in target behaviors of the experimental patients was 10 percent in the controlled setting and 9 percent at home; the control patients changed only 1.5 percent in the experimental setting, and only 2 percent at home.

The spouses in the experimental group showed a median verbal output of 85 responses in the laboratory and 18 responses in the home setting prior to training. After treatment, the median verbal output for these spouses in the experimental situation was 110, and at home it was 27. The median verbal output for the control spouses was 107.5 in the laboratory, and 38 in the home before the investigation began. Following the experiment, the corresponding figures were 90.5 and 38.0. The medians were computed from the total of all verbal responses in all categories.

It was also found that when positive changes occurred in specific target behaviors as a result of treatment, this improvement generalized to other, nontreated categories. Thus, for example, when ***Sentences*** was the target behavior to be increased, patients' increases in sentences were accompanied by improvements in their word and phrase output.

The experimental patients had demonstrated a mean improvement of 6.5 percent on the Functional Communication Profile after they had received speech therapy. Following the conditioning treatment they showed an additional gain of 9.3 percent, despite the fact that nearly all patients had reached a plateau on this measure for at least two months prior to the research.

No significant findings emerged from the administration of the Katz adaptation of the EPPS concerning which spouses make the most effective behavior modifiers.

The investigators noted several advantages in training the spouses of aphasic patients. The spouse, by virtue of the greater amount of time which she spends with the patient than does the speech therapist, is in a position to provide a valuable addition to traditional therapy. (In this study, the spouses, in fact, proved to be better therapists, using behavioral techniques, than the speech therapists.) Families might also be able to save, financially, if spouses can conduct some of the therapy sessions at home. Training spouses rather than simply having them try to help the patients through their own resources assures more effective therapy.

From a psychological viewpoint, inclusion of the spouse in the therapy program gives her a feeling of true involvement and the knowledge that she is helping the patient to recover his lost abilities. Furthermore, by being an integral part of the speech therapy process, the spouse gains greater understanding of the problems involved, and thereby is helped towards realistic expectations and adaptation to the situation. To these may be added the possibility of the spouse utilizing the same general principles and methods for improving other patient behaviors, such as ambulation and upper extremity activities, provided that professional guidance is given.

Goodkin et al.'s use of concurrent response categories is a sound technique with which to evaluate the ongoing verbal behavior of a patient. It can be employed diagnostically, to determine areas of function which are in need of improvement, as a means of evaluating progress in several areas of responding, and as a system with which to assess the effects of new treatment techniques. In particular, with the training of spouses as behavior modifiers, one can study the effects of one person's responses on another person's behavior. Finally, it also makes possible determination of the effect that treatment of one target behavior is having on other responses of the patient.

Two unique procedures employed in this research were the use of teleprompting, whereby the spouse was directed and reinforced for her behaviors, by the experimenter in an adjoining room while she interacted with the patient, and the use of home tape recordings of the verbal interactions between the patients and their spouses. Teleprompting enabled the investigators to build effective training techniques into the spouses' behavior repertoires with more precision and efficiency than would have been the case if they had only reviewed their behaviors with them after each therapy session. The home recordings provided an outside criterion measure to assess the generalization of the effects of the controlled training to a naturalistic environment.

It certainly appears that the results obtained in this experiment warrant further investigation into the area of training family members to therapeutically modify the behaviors of disabled patients.

REFERENCES

Goodkin, R.: Case studies in behavioral research in rehabilitation. *Percept Mot Skills, 23*:171, 1966.

Goodkin, R.: Use of concurrent response categories in evaluating talking behavior in aphasic patients. *Percept Mot Skills, 26*:1035, 1968.

Goodkin, R.: Changes in word production, sentence production and relevance in an aphasic through verbal conditioning. *Behav Res Ther, 7*:93, 1969a.

Goodkin, R.: A procedure for training spouses to improve the functional speech of aphasic patients. Paper presented at the Annual Convention of the American Psychological Association, Washington, 1969b.

Goodkin, R.: The modification of verbal behavior in aphasic subjects. Paper presented at the Annual Convention of the American Psychological Association, Miami Beach, 1970.

Goodkin, R., Diller, L. and Shah, Nandini: Training spouses to improve the functional speech of aphasic patients. In Lahey, B. (Ed.): *The Modification of Language Behavior*. Springfield, Thomas, 1972.

Ince, L. P.: Desensitization with an aphasic patient. *Behav Res Ther, 6*:235, 1968.

Ince, L. P.: Behavior modification with an aphasic man. *Rehab Res Pract Rev, 4*:37, 1973.

Ince, L. P.: *The Rehabilitation Medicine Services*. Springfield, Thomas, 1974.

Ince, L. P. and Rosenberg, D. N.: Modification of articulation in dysarthria. *Arch Phys Med Rehabil, 54*:233, 1973.

Putzer, R. K. and Friedlander, B. Z.: Effects of language status and audio stimulus degradation on preschool children's discriminative listening in an automated operant television game. Paper presented at the Annual Meeting of the American Speech and Hearing Association, New York, 1970.

Roll, D. L.: Modification of nasal resonance in cleft-palate children by informative feedback. *J Appl Behav Anal, 6*:397, 1973.

Taylor, Martha L.: A measurement of functional communication in aphasia. *Arch Phys Med Rehabil, 46*:101, 1964.

Wolpe, J.: *Psychotherapy by Reciprocal Inhibition.* Stanford, Stanford Univ. Press, 1958.

Chapter Six

AUDITORY IMPAIRMENTS

A HEARING LOSS CAN exist either in isolation, or in conjunction with speech and/or language disorders. The latter is true particularly of children when the etiological factor is one of a neurological dysfunction which affects both expressive and receptive aspects of communication.

TESTING

Audiometry

Leibowitz and Drash (1969) dealt with a nine-year-old retarded boy, who had been given several audiometric examinations. Although the results of these tests suggested a hearing loss, the child's lack of functional language and his autistic-like behavior made the results inconclusive.

The investigators decided to establish stimulus control over a conditioned motor response. The response which they selected was the dropping of a poker chip into a can. Initially, they reinforced imitation of this act, and conditioned the behavior without the use of any verbal instructions. Once the response had become established, earphones were placed on the child's head, and loud tones were presented to him. If he dropped the poker chip into the can when a tone was being presented, he received reinforcement. If he performed the response when the tone was not on, a brief time-out period immediately followed, during which he could not receive reinforcement.

Within two 30-minute conditioning sessions, the child learned the required discrimination. An audiometric examination then was administered; the child indicated whether or not he heard the tones presented to him by the examiner by performing the conditioned response.

This technique made it possible to examine the child's hearing effectively, and the results, which revealed a severe sensory-neural hearing loss, were accepted as valid.

The procedure utilized in this study is an application of a basic operant technique requiring a brief time to achieve success. The use of a motor response to indicate auditory discrimination can be extended further. A child may be taught to indicate degrees of hearing by pressing one lever to signal the examiner that a tone or voice sounded loud, and pressing another lever to indicate that the stimulus sounded faint. This is but one example and, in fact, the methodology involved in a study of this nature also can be applied to other perceptual functions such as visual acuity or tactile sensibility, thus being useful for work with individuals who have expressive language impairments.

Sound Discrimination

Friedlander and Whitten (1970) used the PLAYTEST system (see Chapter Four) with an eighteen-month-old infant. The child's mother had contracted rubella during the second month of her pregnancy, and at the age of seven months the child was diagnosed as having a profound hearing loss. She had been fitted with a hearing aid at eleven months of age, but her adaptation to it had not been successful since amplified sound was frightening to her.

The investigators presented the infant with successive pairs of loudness levels by means of nursery rhymes, music and voice selections. The members of each pair of stimuli were presented at different intensity levels, and came through two channels of a "toy," i.e. PLAYTEST console, mounted on the child's crib. Her behavior of playing with the "toy," i.e. selecting channels, was the dependent variable.

From the first day, the infant's behavior clearly could be interpreted in terms of the member of each stimulus pair which she preferred. She was successful in discriminating between sound intensities above 85 db, when they were differentiated by at least 10 db.

The hearing aid was reintroduced during some of the sessions, and the child's listening preference was observed to shift dramatically from highly amplified sound to sounds of low amplification. As the low sounds became audible, the high ones became uncomfortable.

As an additional procedure, the loudness level was held constant at 95 db, and filtered frequencies were regulated across the full range below 1000 Hz and below 500 Hz. It was found that the child could respond selectively to differences in voice and music programs, played with the full range, when they were paired with programs with frequencies above 500 Hz or 1000 Hz filtered out.

The infant now accepted the hearing aid, and her parents reported that she was more aware, by far, of their own voices than she was prior to the study. The entire procedure had been carried out in the child's home, and required seventy-two sessions over a period of two months.

A child with a hearing loss, who could not initially be accurately tested, responded within a brief period of time in such a way that a valid measure could be obtained. Furthermore, because of the methodology employed, her discriminative listening ability became known and she became more responsive to the vocalizations of her family. Finally, a hearing aid, which previously had been rejected by the infant, was accepted and used with a profound positive effect.

* * * * *

In a modification of this procedure, Whitten, Mitsos, Morgan and Friedlander (1970) tested eight children with hearing loss to evaluate their discrimination of loudness levels and filtered frequency spectra.

The ages of the children varied between thirty-nine and eighty-one months, the mean age being sixty-four months. The majority of them had an auditory defect which was the result of prenatal, maternal rubella. The typical hearing loss was one of 70-75 db at 250 Hz, and decreased to a complete lack of response beyond 1500 Hz at a 110 db level. Four normally hearing children also were periodically assessed.

The children were seen individually. Each child was seated before a television display screen on which was projected edited video tape selections from standard children's television programs. The child could manipulate a two-choice, operant switch.

Moving the switch in one direction presented him with one channel or sound, and moving it in the opposite direction opened the other sound channel. The sound intensity levels differed between the two channels, and the child could choose either one to listen to while he watched the television programs. The sessions were of ten minutes or less duration, and the child was free to leave the room at any time, or to remain in the room without operating the switch. (The average performance time of the group at the task was 85 percent of the total time spent in the room.)

Phase	*Preschool Population*	*Stimulus Properties*		*Total Response Output*	*Discrimination*	*Time or Task*
		Channel I	Channel II			
1	5 Clinicals/HA*	85 dB/Video	0/0	2577 Seconds	Positive	89%
2	5 Clinicals/HA	85 dB/Video	0/Video	2255	Positive	75
3	5 Clinicals/HA	85 dB/Video	65 dB/Video	2579	Positive	86
4	5 Clinicals/HA	85 dB/Video	75 dB/Video	2628	Positive	88
5	5 Clinicals/HA	85 dB/Video	80 dB/Video	2586	Positive	86
6	8 Clinicals/HA	75 dB/Video	65 dB/Video	3616	Positive	79
7	4 Normals	75 dB/Video	65 dB/Video	2075	Negative	87
8	8 Clinicals/HA	80 dB<500 Hz./ Video	80 dB Normal/ Video	4149	Negative	88
9	8 Clinicals/HA	80 dB-1000 Hz./ Video	80 dB Normal/ Video	3995	Mixed	90
				26,460		Mn 85%

*HA = Hearing Aids

Table 6-I Selection of preferred soundtracks in a TV game. From Whitten, D. A., Mitsos, S. B., Morgan, Marion T. and Friedlander, B. Z.: Effects of loudness and sound spectrum on hearing impaired preschool children's operant selection of preferred soundtrack in an automated videotape TV game. Paper presented at the Annual Meeting of the American Speech and Hearing Association, New York, 1970.

Reproduced with the permission of the senior author and the American Speech and Hearing Association.

Table 6-I shows that the hearing-impaired children consistently were able to discriminate differences in sound level as fine as five db in the 80 to 85 db range, and 10 db in the 65 to 75 db range. Only two of the children failed to make these discriminations well. There was a tendency from phase to phase, toward increased length of average response duration.

The test results were less conclusive for filtered frequencies. The group generally could not distinguish between a normal sound track and one which excluded frequencies above 500 Hz.

When the sound tract was filtered above 1000 Hz, some children preferred the normal sound track while others chose the filtered channel to listen to.

A procedure such as the one employed in this investigation makes it possible not only to test a child's discriminative hearing ability, but to do so in a manner which is pleasant and nonaversive for the child. Thus, much important information concerning a patient's auditory capacity, which will be valuable for therapy and training, can be obtained.

TRAINING

It is well known that persons who are born deaf usually have some type or types of speech dysfunction. Inability to hear the sounds which others make, or to receive feedback from their own vocalizations, presents a serious handicap which interferes with the development of normal voice quality. The genesis of normal vocal pitch or frequency is important in the speech of the deaf since correct speech production depends at least partially on an appropriate distribution of vocal energy.

The spacing of components of complex voiced speech sounds is related directly to the fundamental vocal frequency. Therefore, high-pitched voices tend to provide an inadequate energy distribution for speech, since there are an inadequate number of harmonics available for the optimal production of speech sounds. This results in a loss of the speaker's intelligibility.

Modification of Vocal Impairments

In an attempt to bring the fundamental vocal frequency within limits appropriate to the age and sex of the speaker, Holbrook and Meador (1969) developed an apparatus called FLORIDA®, which is an acronym for Frequency Lowering Or Raising Intensity Determining Apparatus (see also Holbrook and Crawford, 1970a).

With this equipment, the subject is seated before a microphone, which is placed approximately six inches below and in front of his chin. A red light and a white light are located within his visual periphery. When he speaks, the signal from the microphone is relayed to an amplifier, and the amplified sound is fed into a tape recorder for storage and future analysis. The amplified signal also is fed into a variable electronic band pass filter system with a 72 db/octave attenuator slope, and into an overload circuit within a programmer unit. The signal which is passed by the filter feeds into a target circuit and a monitor oscilloscope. The filter can be adjusted to pass a band of vocal frequencies which are appropriate for the subject's sex and age. The target unit signals the subject when he is emitting an appropriate range of fundamental vocal frequencies. Thus, the subject need not speak monotonically, but with normal fluctuations of voice frequency. These will activate the target circuit, closing a relay which turns on the white light. This signals correct responding to the subject and energizes a timer which measures the duration of on-target responses per trial.

The overload circuit signals the subject that he is speaking too loudly. It receives the unfiltered sound, shutting off the white light and the timer, and turning on the red light.

The oscilloscope receives the output of the filter on one axis, and the output of an oscillator on the other axis. A frequency counter, connected in parallel with the oscillator, assures the accuracy of the oscillator settings. The oscilloscope is used by the experimenter for monitoring purposes, displaying a Lissajous figure in the form of a circle when the filtered fundamental is the same frequency as that of the oscillator. The amplitude of the figure is at maximum when the oscillator frequency is at the center of the band pass filter, thus providing the experimenter with a verification of the accuracy of the filter settings.

The apparatus reinforces appropriate fundamental vocal frequency while it simultaneously controls excessive intensity. FLORIDA may be used with both children and adults.

Holbrook and Crawford (1970b) improved the vocal performance of four deaf persons, aged twenty-eight to forty-eight years. All of the subjects had poor control of fundamental vocal frequency and intensity, and all had abnormally high levels of vocal pitch. The goal of the study was to bring their frequency levels down to normal.

Before initiating modification procedures, baseline data were collected for all subjects. Each subject read a passage within four-minute trials. The voice controller was adjusted to measure the duration of responding within the frequency region of the subject's voice, which was judged to be optimal for his age, sex, and usual vocal level and range. Each subject read the passage until baseline stability had occurred. Stability was defined as the ninth trial duration falling within the range of the preceding eight trials. The subjects were told only to read the passage in such a way that the white light would remain on and the red light would remain off.

Following the baseline phase, the subjects received positive reinforcement, i.e. the white light, for vocal frequencies appropriate to the parameters to which the voice controller had been adjusted. The subject's vocal behavior was shaped by successive approximations. The limits of the frequency regions which activated the voice controller were narrowed gradually. Reinforcement was delivered on an FR1 schedule until the subjects achieved a high rate of responding within the desired frequency range.

Once the conditioned responses had stabilized, an extinction period was introduced, during which the conditioning lights were inoperative.

After the extinction trials, the conditioned response was reinstated, with the lights being available again contingent upon appropriate responding.

Finally, variable interval schedules of reinforcement were substituted for the continuous reinforcement schedule. These varied from having a mean of six seconds, to having a mean of 140 seconds, and were, consecutively, VI6, VI12, VI20, VI28, VI41, VI60, VI90, VI105, VI125 and VI140. The reinforcement period consisted of ten seconds during which the conditioning lights were available.

Eight 4-minute trials were conducted daily, four days per week for seven weeks.

Three women and one male subject took part in the study. Baseline data indicated that the modal pitch level for the male was 260 Hz. The modal pitch levels for the female subjects were 470 Hz, 300 Hz and 300 Hz. Following conditioning, the modal pitch levels had been changed to 130 Hz for the male subject, a reduction of one octave; 210 Hz, for one of the female subjects, a reduction of more than one octave; and 225 Hz for the other two females.

During extinction, the pitch levels of the subjects rose to slightly above those of the conditioning phase, but these levels were still well below baseline frequencies. The variable interval schedules of reinforcement were successful in maintaining the conditioned behavior for relatively long periods of time.

The subjects were followed up for three months after the experiment had been terminated. Two of the participants had maintained their conditioned responses and two had returned to pitch levels which were midway between their baseline and conditioning levels.

* * * * *

Holbrook also employed FLORIDA with deaf school-age children. Three children, aged seven, nine, and eleven years, were selected for the study because they had abnormally high levels of vocal pitch. Each child read passages appropriate to his academic level. Conditioning took place during eight 30-second trials per day for a period of six weeks.

At the end of the treatment period, the fundamental vocal frequency of each child had been modified dramatically. The seven-year-old child had an initial baseline mode of 450 Hz, and conditioning reduced it to a mode of 350 Hz. The nine-year-old had a baseline fundamental modal frequency of 510 Hz, which was lowered to 310 Hz by the conditioning procedure. The eleven-year-old began the study at a modal frequency of 450 Hz, and this was decreased to a mode of 370 Hz.

* * * * *

These procedures also were successful with preschool children, using food as a reinforcer (Holbrook, 1970), but most interesting of all, perhaps, was the use of FLORIDA with a fifteen-month-old, deaf baby girl (Holbrook, 1971).

Because of the inappropriateness of light as a reinforcer for so young a patient, food was used as the reward. A feeder which was activated by the voice-controlling apparatus was mounted immediately in front of the infant. When the baby's vocal pitch and intensity fell within the limits determined by the experimenter, the feeder was activated and food was presented to her. A white light, mounted on the front of the feeder, provided an additional cue. The baby's teacher was present in the experimental room at all times, and initially reinforced the baby at the end of each thirty-second trial. The teacher repeatedly demonstrated to her that her voice would result in activation of the feeder. After ten demonstrations, the baby began to vocalize, thus operating the feeder herself.

Ten 30-second trials were conducted per day during the experimental period.

Initially, the infant's vocal frequency varied between 800 Hz and 1200 Hz. Gradually the limits were narrowed, and after ten weeks of conditioning her pitch level was between 300 Hz and 400 Hz, with good vocal quality. At first, her filter band pass was at 500-1500 Hz, so that her high-pitched voice could be reinforced. Then the frequence range of the filters was lowered so that by the tenth week of the study the filters were set to pass frequencies of 200-400 Hz, and the infant used a pitch level of 300 Hz to activate the feeder. This behavior generalized to her home, and her parents reported that she used the lowered pitch level there too.

* * * * *

Holbrook and Crawford (1970b) were able to modify hypernasality in three deaf adults by making reinforcement, in the form of white light, contingent upon nonnasal tones, and punishment, delivered as red light, contingent upon nasal responses.

A transducer, consisting of a phonograph cartridge with a weighted needle, was taped to each subject's nose. Upon nasal emissions, the tissues of the nose were set into vibration, and the inertia of the phonograph needle caused a voltage to be developed within the cartridge which then was amplified and closed the punishment relay.

Two stop clocks were employed, one accumulating the duration of oral, nonnasal responses during a three-minute trial period, and the other clock accumulating the duration of hypernasal responses. As one clock was activated, the other was deactivated.

Following a baseline period, the subjects were informed that the white light indicated "good" performance, while the red light signalled that they were doing something wrong. The subjects read from a passage which contained no nasal sounds, and were instructed to try to keep the white light on and the red light off.

The results can briefly be summarized by stating that the oral durations of the subjects' responses significantly increased while their nasal durations markedly and dramatically decreased. Extinction trials did not extinguish the conditioned behavior.

The work of Holbrook and his associates clearly demonstrates the feasibility of an operant approach to training the deaf to speak more normally. The advantages of using automated apparatus are obvious. Speech is deemed abnormal in terms of the listener. When the listener pays more attention to the characteristics of the speech sounds than to the content of what is being said, the speaker's vocalizations are considered to be impaired. However, in a research study it often is very difficult to make rapid decisions concerning the intelligibility of a subject so that reinforcement can be delivered appropriately. By knowing the frequency range of normal speech, thus predetermining the desired responses, and by regulating automated equipment to respond to them, Holbrook overcame this difficulty. The experimenters did not have to attend constantly to the subjects, nor was the possibility of human error a variable to contend with since the correct contingencies were automatically programmed.

Shaping played an important role in these investigations, particularly in the work with the deaf adults who had been speaking abnormally for many years. It could not be expected that they would respond immediately in the appropriate manner if the reinforcement requirement was speech within a narrow frequency range. Thus, reinforcement initially was made contingent upon vocalizations to which they were habituated and the range then was gradually narrowed to normal pitch levels. Had the experimenters begun with a stringent criterion for reinforcement, it is unlikely that the same successful results would have been achieved.

There is great promise in the fact that not only adults, but deaf children and even infants can be trained in this way. The addition of food as a reinforcer was significant with the preschool children and the baby girl, since small children seldom are impressed with adult goals and thus often require different motivations. It should also be noted that in the study conducted with the fifteen-month-old baby, only ten 30-second trials per day were attempted. An infant's attention span is very short. Therefore, extended experimental time, while more convenient for the researcher, would have made the situation aversive for the subject in addition to the probability that much of the data would have been meaningless after a brief number of trials.

The modification of hypernasality demonstrated that more than one type of speech dysfunction can be treated with the FLORIDA system, or with similar automated apparatus. Perhaps impairments of rate and articulation, breathiness, and other vocal characteristics can also be modified with such behavioral methods.

Speech Habilitation

A hearing loss alone presents serious problems, both for the affected individual and to those engaged in the therapeutic process. These problems become multiplied when they are compounded by other disorders, such as autism, mental retardation, motoric involvement, or blindness, to name but a few possible additional complications. Often, factors other then the auditory impairment must be dealt with simultaneously, or even prior to, working with the target behaviors.

This point is illustrated by the study of Benassi and Benassi (1973), in which they treated a six-year-old male with rubella syndrome who was diagnosed as being cerebral palsied, mentally retarded and deaf. Audiological examinations revealed a severe, bilateral, sensory-neural hearing loss.

As a consequence of the child's cerebral dysfunction, he was unable to ambulate or sit unsupported for any length of time. Therefore, he was placed in either a prone or supine position, or was strapped into a special chair. He had been fitted with a bilateral low frequency emphasis hearing aid so as to provide him with some degree of auditory stimulation.

The patient's behavior consisted, primarily, of self-stimulation activities such as gazing at lights through his fingers, and pressing on his eye while looking at lights. He only looked at people rarely, and he would not look at other objects for extended periods of time. Occasionally, he would look at or grab others, and frequently he engaged in crying, head banging and arm biting for relatively lengthy intervals. The child had no functional language, and vocalized only two consonant sounds and a few vowel sounds.

The treatment procedure involved three main phases and required a total of fifty-two sessions, each session varying between fifteen and thirty minutes in duration. The patient was seen twice per week for the first thirty sessions, and three times per week for the remaining twenty-one sessions.

Phase I (Sessions 1-6) — The target behavior in this initial phase was designated as "looking at the experimenter's face." The child was placed on the floor in a supine position. A cardboard box was fitted over him so that the walls of the box were behind and to the sides of his head, thereby limiting his visual field. He was able to see only the walls of the box and what was straight up, i.e. the experimenter's face, the ceiling and the lights. Reinforcement, in the form of food, was given each time the child looked at the experimenter's face. Simultaneous with the delivery of food, the experimenter rubbed the child's face and smiled at him.

Phase II (Sessions 7-13) — Once the target behavior of the preceding phase had been established, reinforcement was given to the child only for looking at the experimenter's face for at least five seconds. Responses of less than five seconds duration were recorded but not rewarded.

Phase III (Sessions 14-52) — After the child's behavior of looking at the experimenter for five seconds or longer had been conditioned, she began to vocalize the sound "ah" as soon as he looked at her, and maintained the sound for five seconds.

If the patient vocalized during that time, he received reinforcement. This procedure continued for twenty-three sessions.

As the child's vocalizations came under the control of the experimenter's verbal cues, his disruptive behaviors, which had been reduced to a minimum at the beginning of the study, began to increase in frequency. He spent a considerable part of the time trying to get out of the cardboard box. He then was placed in a tilt chair, with the box removed, and was tilted to an angle of 20 degrees with no restrictions on his visual field. The disruptive behaviors rapidly extinguished, and discriminative vocalization was reinstated to a high frequency of occurrence. After a few sessions, he was placed in the special restraining chair with no resultant deleterious effects on his responding.

From Sessions 37 to 45, reinforcement was delivered according to an FR2 schedule and then, for the remainder of the study, the schedule was switched to a VR2 program.

Throughout the study, whenever the patient engaged in disruptive behaviors, the experimenter responded by turning her body away from him until they ceased.

The data for the rate of attention responses for each experimental session are presented in Table 6-II. It can be seen that the child acquired the target behavior and maintained it throughout the study. The percentage column of the table indicates that nearly all of his responses were of five seconds duration or longer. In addition, the child's mother, physical therapist, and occupational therapist all reported that his behavior had generalized to the home and other therapy situations.

The percentage of times that the child vocalized after the experimenter's prompt are reported in Figure 6-1, beginning with Session 19. While discriminated vocalization was developed rapidly under conditions of continuous reinforcement it began to deteriorate as inappropriate behaviors increased in frequency. In the twenty-fourth session, the child was placed in the tilt chair, and this resulted in increased discriminative vocalizing.

It is interesting that the response percentages were not greatly affected by the change to FR2 and VR2 reinforcement schedules. The investigators felt that by decreasing the density of reinforcement while maintaining correct responses at a high level, the

Session no.	Total	5 sec or more	less than 5 sec.	% 5 sec/more to total
1	1.50			
2	2.20			
3	2.70			
4	1.86			
5	1.70			
6	1.88			
7	2.30	1.15	1.15	50
8	3.05	1.85	1.20	61
9	1.65	0.95	0.70	58
10	1.90	1.25	0.65	66
11	1.95	1.35	0.60	69
12	1.20	0.84	0.36	70
13	1.90	1.45	0.45	76
14	2.20	1.97	0.23	89
15	1.40	1.13	0.27	81
16	1.56	1.36	0.20	87
17	1.90	1.85	0.05	97
18	2.20	1.93	0.27	88
19	0.73	0.67	0.06	91
20	0.93	0.80	0.13	86
21	0.50	0.37	0.13	73
22	0.93	0.63	0.30	68
23	0.50	0.30	0.20	60
24	1.00	0.95	0.05	95
25	0.95	0.90	0.05	95
26	1.52	1.48	0.04	97
27	0.84	0.84	0.00	100
28	1.73	1.66	0.07	96
29	1.50	1.40	0.10	93
30	1.68	1.52	0.16	90
31	1.30	1.25	0.05	96
32	1.29	1.23	0.06	95
33	1.70	1.60	0.10	94
34	1.73	1.66	0.07	96
35	1.60	1.45	0.15	91
36	2.50	2.31	0.19	93
37	1.10	1.00	0.10	91
38	1.70	1.64	0.06	97
39	1.40	1.13	0.27	81
40	1.64	1.52	0.12	93
41	1.09	0.95	0.14	88
42	1.60	1.45	0.15	91
43	1.70	1.60	0.10	94
44	1.61	1.55	0.06	97
45	1.47	1.30	0.17	88
46	1.47	1.34	0.13	91
47	1.80	1.60	0.20	88
48	1.60	1.40	0.20	87
49	1.90	1.85	0.05	97
50	0.90	0.75	0.15	83
51	1.65	1.50	0.15	91
52	1.60	1.45	0.15	91

Table 6-II Rate of attention responses (per minute) and percentage of five seconds or more responses to total responses. From Benassi, Barbara J. and Benassi, V. A.: Behavioral strategies for a deaf and cerebral palsied child. *J Communic Dis, 6*:165, 1973.

Reproduced with the permission of the authors and the North-Holland Publishing Company, Amsterdam, Netherlands.

experimental sessions were made to more closely resemble the subject's natural environment, wherein reinforcement would not follow each time certain behaviors are performed.

An additional finding was that the disruptive behaviors of eye pressing, arm biting, head banging, etc., which had existed at a high frequency prior to the study, decreased during the first few sessions and remained at near zero, with few exceptions, for the remainder of the program.

Prior to the conditioning program, many of those who had contact with the patient had set limited and restricted goals for

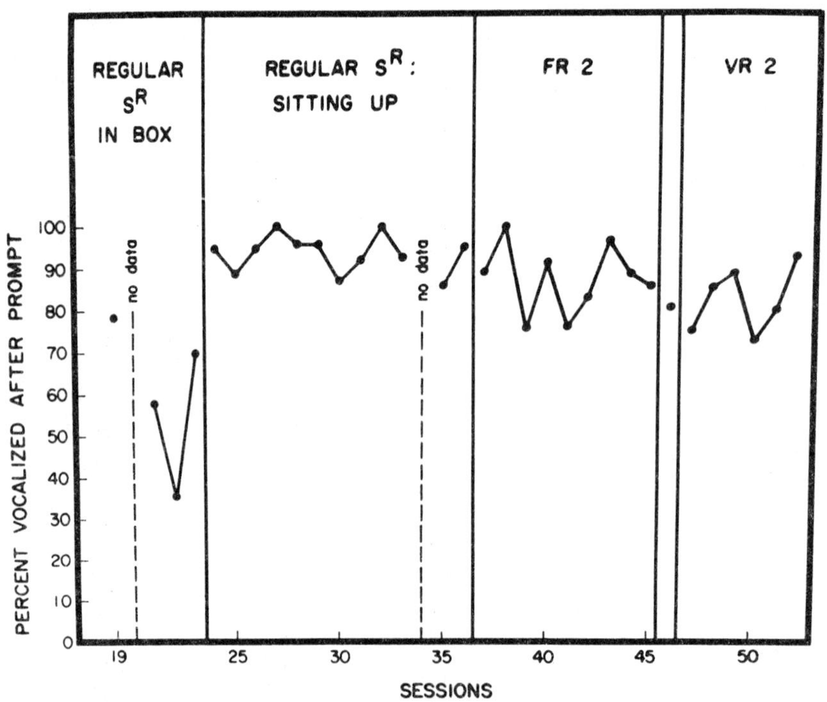

Figure 6-1 Percentage of times that *S* vocalized after *E*'s prompt (by session). S_R = reinforcement. From Benassi, Barbara J. and Benassi, V. A.: Behavioral strategies for a deaf and cerebral palsied child. *J Communic Dis, 6*:165, 1973.

Reproduced with the permission of the authors and the North-Holland Publishing Company, Amsterdam, Netherlands.

him because of their belief that he did not possess adequate learning ability. Although a cursory evaluation might lead to such a conclusion, based upon the fact that not only was the child deaf and cerebral palsied but mentally defective as well, conceptions of this nature are not plausible from a behavioral viewpoint.

The investigators point out that the major limitations of this type of case lie in the therapist's ability to develop and implement effective techniques. As mentioned previously in this volume, one never should enter into a program with preconceived ideas concerning the capacity of the subjects. Not only will this restrict the number and kinds of procedures attempted, but will bias the investigator towards certain results and conclusions. In Benassi's study, the goals were three-fold: reducing disruptive behavior, gaining attention, and instating vocalization; success was achieved with each one, although only to a limited extent for the last-named, because the child's family moved from the vicinity. However, based upon the gains which were made, it appears plausible that, had the behavior modification program continued, the patient would have learned at least some functional language.

BEHAVIOR PROBLEMS OF THE DEAF

Many children with a hearing loss exhibit a variety of maladaptive behaviors. Some of these problems result from the child's sensory loss, which limits his environment and his ability to respond to it appropriately, others stem from the young age factor, and still others may be attributable to the inexperience or naivete of the parents. While it is, of course, possible to conduct behavior therapy with the child, when one considers that such therapy typically involves only a few hours of a child's total waking time, at best, this approach appears to be an uneconomical one. Instead, it seems more profitable to work with the child's parents, those people with whom the child spends the greatest proportion of his days.

Mira (1972) reported on several cases of behavior problems, among children who were hard of hearing, which she treated in this manner.

A common problem faced by parents of hearing-impaired children is their inability to extend vocal control of the child over distance. Being unable to remotely signal a child verbally is both inconvenient and a source of fear, since the child can get lost in crowds or be endangered by automotive vehicles because he cannot hear their sounds or the shouted warnings of his parents.

Such a problem is represented by the case of a three and one-half-year-old boy, with a mild hearing loss, who ran away from his mother so frequently that the behavior became life-threatening.

In order to deal with this, the boy's mother was assigned two behavior modification projects to carry out. The first one involved teaching the child to play within established boundaries. During a two-week baseline period, his mother instructed him to play within an area bounded by adjacent driveways. No other restraints were placed upon him, and a record was kept of the rate at which he turned back into the play area when he had gone to either boundary. His turn-back rate during this period was zero; once he crossed a boundary he did not return to the play area.

In the next phase, the child's mother gave him a gumdrop each time he turned back at the boundary. If he crossed over a boundary, he was taken to his room for ten minutes. To "prime" correct behavior, his mother pushed him on his tricycle, to the boundary, turned him around, smiled, and placed a gumdrop in his mouth.

This procedure resulted in a median turn-back rate of .3 responses per minute. Simultaneously, boundary crossing dropped to zero. After fifteen days, candy was no longer given, at the child's request, but turn-backs remained at nearly the same level, and boundary crossings were maintained at zero. Figure 6-2 presents the data. ("Chart only" refers to the baseline period.)

The second project was designed to teach the child to remain with his mother rather than run away from her when they left the home. Baseline rates showed a median of eight to nine runaways per day.

The supermarket was selected as the primary training site. The child's mother held him by the hand and walked to the gum machine upon entering the store. She bought one piece of gum,

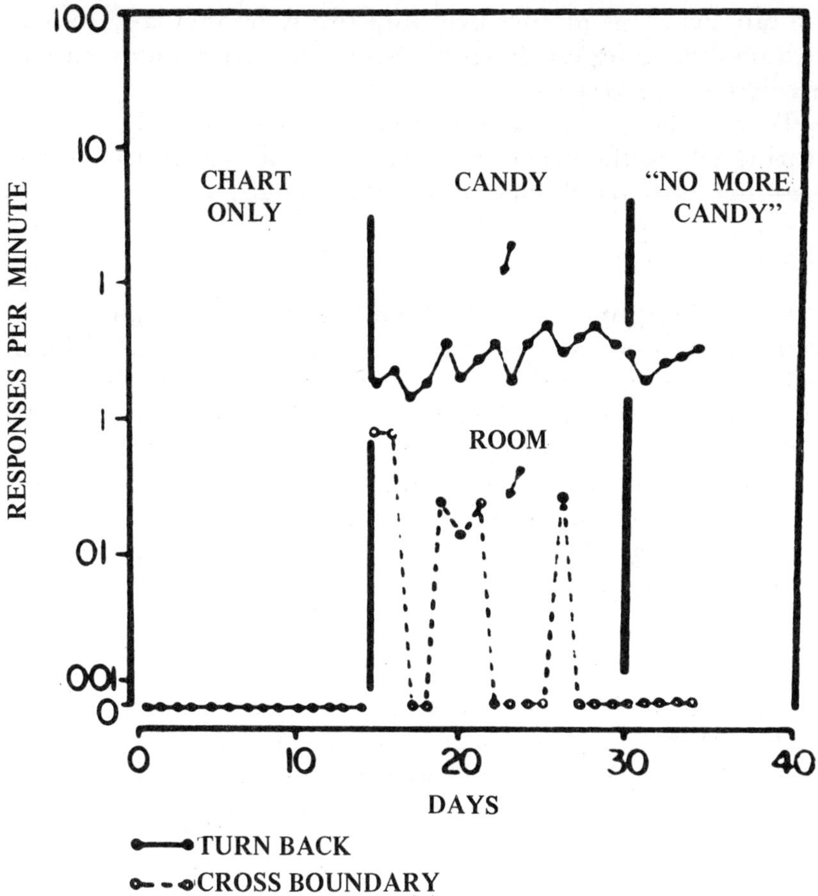

Figure 6-2 Deceleration of boundary crossing by reinforcement with candy. From Mira, Mary: Behavior modification applied to training young deaf children. *Except Child, 39*:225, 1972.

Reproduced with the permission of the author and The Council for Exceptional Children.

released his hand, walked a few steps, turned to him, and said, "Good. You stayed with me," and gave him the gum. Each successive day, she required that he walk with her a little further in order to receive the gum until, by the end of three weeks, he had to remain with her until they left the store to receive the reinforcer. If he ran away, his mother held him firmly by the hand for two minutes. Begging for the gum resulted in two minutes without receiving his mother's attention.

During the first week of this project, there were several days during which there were no runaways, and within five weeks, running away had been eliminated entirely.

* * * * *

Child discipline, often a difficult matter for any parent, becomes even more of a problem for the parents of a deaf child. In addition to the complications presented in the home, difficulties in child management frequently have to be dealt with if speech and language training programs are to be successful. It commonly is found that once undesirable behaviors have been eliminated in the home environment, appropriate behaviors generalize to other settings. Therefore, the initial task of modifying a child's maladaptive responses is the parents'.

* * * * *

A little girl, whose mother Mira worked with, exhibited the act of hitting her mother whenever she tried to discipline her. In response, her mother would pout, feign dismay, and shake her finger at the child. The child's teacher, however, encouraged the mother to expect normal social behavior, and a behavior modification approach was implemented.

Over a ten-day period, baseline measures were made. The child's mother recorded three to four hits per day, with only one day during which no hits occurred. Thereafter, each time she was hit by her daughter, the mother turned her back and walked away for five minutes, regardless of what she and the child were doing at the time.

Within one week, the rate of hitting declined, and by the fourth week it had been reduced to zero. A follow-up three months later revealed that the hitting behavior had not returned, nor had any other undesirable response been substituted.

* * * * *

Another discipline problem frequently encountered among hearing-impaired children is marked negativism.

Two preschool children, a boy and a girl, met directions with head shakes, stamping of the feet, and vehement "No"s. If their mothers insisted, the children typically resorted to temper tantrums. The little girl exhibited a baseline median rate of one negative behavior every ten minutes of observation, and the boy had a median baseline frequency of four negative acts per ten-minute period.

Both parents employed a time-out procedure to eliminate these responses. When the child reacted negatively, the mother led him to his room, indicating that when he did such a thing he could not keep on playing or remain outside with his parents. The child had to remain in the room for a predetermined interval, usually ten minutes in length. When the designated time period had elapsed, if the tantrum was still ongoing, the time-in-the-room period was extended until the child was quiet for two minutes. The room had neither toys with which to play nor people with whom to interact.

By the second week, the little girl's negative responses had been reduced. The results were achieved even more rapidly with the boy. A followup 100 days later showed that these behaviors had not returned. The data are presented in Figure 6-3.

* * * * *

The final problem to be discussed here is the refusal of a hard-of-hearing child to wear a required hearing aid.

Mira saw a three-and one-half-year-old child who refused to wear his new hearing aid except during training sessions.

His mother was instructed to allow him to watch his favorite television programs, or to play his record player once each day if he wore the aid for a specified period of time.

Within one week, she was able to increase the length of time the child wore the device.

Then, the contingencies were altered from permitting him to watch television or play the record player once each day, to allowing these activities every three hours, providing that the child

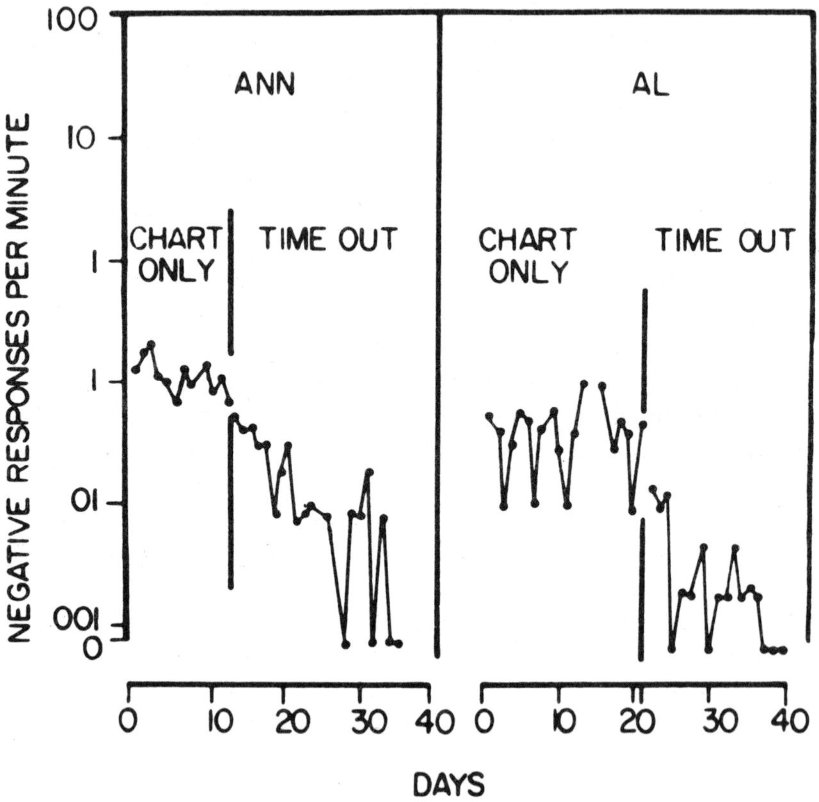

Figure 6-3 Deceleration of negative behavior by time-out procedures. From Mira, Mary: Behavior modification applied to training young deaf children. *Except Child, 39*:225, 1972.

had worn the hearing aid during the previous three hours. This resulted in his wearing the aid for the entire day.

These examples all serve to illustrate that operant-based child management procedures can successfully alleviate a variety of problems which can interfere with a hearing impaired child's development of communication. The reader must be struck by the simplicity of the methods involved, yet it is their very simplicity which makes them so amenable to application by parents, therapists and special educators.

It is uneconomical for the behavioral scientist to spend his time with each patient because the techniques which he uses are so complex that only he can implement them. A far more efficient approach is to train others, particularly those with whom the patient spends the most time, to carry out the procedures. In this way, parents can manage their own children in their natural environments, and therapists and teachers can utilize the methods with the many children with whom they come into contact daily. The fact that this can be easily done represents one of the major advantages of a behavior modification approach.

REFERENCES

Benassi, Barbara J. and Benassi, V. A.: Behavioral strategies for a deaf and cerebral palsied child. *J Communic Dis, 6*:165, 1973.

Friedlander, B. Z. and Whitten, D. A.: Effects of regulated loudness and sound frequency on an 18-month-old "deaf" infant's discriminative self-selected listening with an automated operant game in the home. Paper presented at the Annual Meeting of the American Speech and Hearing Association, New York, 1970.

Holbrook, A.: Modification of speech behaviors with pre-school deaf children by means of spectrum control. *AOEHI Bull, 1*:60, 1970.

Holbrook, A.: Procedures for conditioning deaf infants with speech teaching machines. Paper presented to the European Association for Special Education, Norrkoping, Sweden, 1971.

Holbrook, A. and Crawford, Gladys H.: Modifications of vocal frequency and intensity in the speech of the deaf. *Volta Rev, 72*:492, 1970a.

Holbrook, A. and Crawford, Gladys H.: Modification of speech behavior in the speech of the deaf. Paper presented at the Conference of Executives of American Schools for the Deaf, St. Augustine, 1970b.

Holbrook, A. and Meador, M. M.: A device for automatic modification of vocal frequency and intensity. *South Speech J, 35*:154, 1969.

Leibowitz, J. M. and Drash, P. W.: Use of an operant technique as an adjunct in testing auditory discrimination in a non-verbal retarded child. Paper presented at the Annual Convention of the Eastern Psychological Association, Philadelphia, 1969.

Mira, Mary: Behavior modification applied to training young deaf children. *Except Child, 39*:225, 1972.

Whitten, D. A., Mitsos, S. B., Morgan, Marion T. and Friedlander, B. Z.: Effects of loudness and sound spectrum on hearing impaired preschool children's operant selection of preferred soundtrack in an automated videotape TV game. Paper presented at the Annual Meeting of the American Speech and Hearing Association, New York, 1970.

SECTION IV

THE MODIFICATION OF BEHAVIORAL AND MANAGEMENT PROBLEMS

INTRODUCTION

UNLIKE PATIENTS IN an acute hospital, those who are institutionalized for rehabilitation remain in the hospital for relatively long periods of time. Because of the nature and the severity of their physical disabilities, it is unlikely that a rehabilitation program designed to restore the patient to maximal capability will take less than three or four months of intensive therapeutic efforts. Frequently, an even lengthier stay is required if an individual is to learn to function satisfactorily within the limitations imposed upon him by his disability. When chronic, progressive diseases such as multiple sclerosis and muscular dystrophy are considered, institutionalization can become a matter of years. Thus, the patient population of these settings tends to become relatively stable, and to form a community within the hospital which resembles, in many respects, the general community at large.

When this occurs, one finds many of the same problems which exist in society also existing within the hospital population. These range from the more serious ones, such as hostility with aggressive acting-out, drug abuse, alcohol intoxication and theft, to "in-group" formations, negativism, lack of motivation, uncooperative behavior, complaining and poor self-care, plus a host of other major and minor difficulties.

With the advent of the application of behavior modification methodology in the rehabilitation field, the psychologist has become far more effective in dealing with behavioral and management problems. This section discusses a variety of such problems and their resolution by behavioral procedures.

Chapter Seven

PROBLEMS OF MOTIVATION

LACK OF MOTIVATION is a serious problem in rehabilitation. To those who are unfamiliar with disabled patients, it might seem that any individual whose daily functioning has been limited severely by a physical disability would be highly motivated to regain lost function and become as independent in his daily activities as possible. Such an individual would be expected to attend all therapy classes regularly and punctually, work hard during his therapy sessions, and try to practice in other areas of the hospital what he has learned from his therapists.

Professionals working in the rehabilitation field know that this is not the case. There are, of course, many patients who do conform to those expectations, but there are also many who do not. A number of patients either attend their prescribed therapy sessions on an irregular basis, or do not attend them at all. Some will attend, but arrive late for their appointments and perform the various required tasks and exercises in a lackadaisical manner. Many follow the therapist's instructions while in class, but seldom or never attempt to use their abilities on their wards or floors, or at home. Others resist all attempts at therapy, presenting various and numerous excuses as to why they "cannot" participate in their program.

There are several reasons for lack of motivation among rehabilitation patients, and the interested reader can consult Ince (1974) for a discussion of this general topic. This chapter focusses on the behavioral approach to some of the motivation problems of the hospitalized disabled.

PERSISTENCE AT A TASK

Meyerson, Kerr and Michael (1967) worked with an eighteen-year-old, quadriplegic man two years after an automobile accident had resulted in impairments of binocular vision, speech, memory, attention span and muscular coordination. He was wheelchair-bound, and had severe tremors of the upper extremities.

The patient's occupational therapist had selected typing as a task which was interesting, and useful in improving his eye-hand coordination. The problem was that although the patient verbally expressed the desire to learn to type, he really did not attend to the task. His behavior consisted of typing a few letters, stopping, and calling for the therapist with a question or a complaint. At times, he stopped his work and waited for her to approach him to inquire as to why he was not typing. Because of this behavior, which also interfered with the therapist's functioning with other patients, he was considered to be unmotivated, and to have reached a plateau in his ability. Thus, the therapist felt that he should be discharged from the hospital.

The psychologists' observations of the patient revealed that he never worked for longer than seven minutes at a time before calling for the therapist's attention. She always responded by going to him, answering his question or complaint, and chatting with him briefly before coaxing him to resume his work. It appeared, therefore, that the therapist actually was reinforcing the undesirable behavior of the patient. He enjoyed talking with her more than he liked typing. Since the therapist invariably responded to his demands, the patient was in control of the situation.

The psychologists decided that the goals of a behavior modification program should be the following: typing for at least thirty minutes without calling for the therapist's attention; increasing work output in terms of number of lines typed; and improving typing accuracy.

In order to achieve these aims, two changes were made in the therapy situation. First, the typewriter and the patient were moved from the large occupational therapy area where the unmotivated behavior had been reinforced, to a smaller, more isolated room. This was done both to weaken the past behavior by introducing new discriminative stimuli, and to decrease response alternatives that were made possible by the presence and activities of other people. Second, social reinforcement was made contingent upon typing behavior. Following each thirty-minute session during which the patient typed more lines than during the previous session, he was given five minutes of social interaction on the "man-to-man" basis. The topics discussed were those of masculine interest, including athletics, automobiles, etc. Two sessions were conducted per week.

The task was sufficiently difficult for the patient so that if he stopped typing for several minutes during the session it was impossible for him to meet the criterion for reinforcement. When he did not exceed the previous session's output he did not receive the social reinforcement.

In addition, to avoid demands for attention, reinforcement was given for smaller units of work. Approximately every five minutes the experimenter entered the room, estimated the number of words typed, and if the patient's output appeared to be greater than that of the previous period, the experimenter praised him and then left the room.

After only one thirty-minute session, in which the variable interval reinforcement was given and demands for attention were ignored, the patient no longer attempted to converse with the experimenter during the work period. Following the ninth session, the patient requested that the experimenter no longer enter the room during the period since this slowed down his work output.

From the second to the twelfth session, the patient attended to the task for the entire thirty minutes without stopping his typing or calling for the therapist. His typing rate increased at this time from five lines in the first session to twelve lines by the twelfth session, while his errors concurrently decreased from three per line to a mean of one-half error per line.

From the thirteenth through the fifteenth sessions, the duration of typing increased to sixty minutes, with but a single five-minute reinforcement interval after thirty minutes. The patient's attention to the task was maintained without a reduction of lines typed or an increase in errors.

The patient appeared motivated, and it was clear that even further gains could be made if his therapist, who now took over his treatment, maintained the reinforcement contingencies.

In their determination of how to treat the problem presented by this patient, the investigators asked four basic questions.

1. What is the desirable behavior? This is of primary consideration in any study. It is not sufficient simply to state that a patient should "do more," or "show more interest and motivation." The precise behavior(s) to be increased or instated must clearly be specified.

2. What is the criterion for success? This question must be answered in terms of frequency of specified behaviors, amount of time spent engaged in those behaviors, and speed and/or accuracy of performance. Based upon these, the goals for improved responding were selected.

3. What behavior must be modified? That is, which behaviors are to be generated or increased, and which are to be extinguished? If desirable and undesirable behaviors are incompatible, the expectation is that reinforcing the former will maintain them. However, in rehabilitation, where therapists have been trained to respond to the needs of their patients, they may reinforce undesirable behaviors as well as those which they are trying to increase or maintain.

In the study just described, the therapist did give attention for typing, but also gave it for nontyping behavior as well. Thus, she was maintaining both behaviors.

It is important to extinguish incompatible behaviors if relearning is to occur, particularly when the desired behaviors are present in at least minimal strength. In cases of new learning, when the desired responses are not present, techniques other than extinction for modifying behavior must be considered.

4. What will serve as a reinforcer? When it is not known what is reinforcing for a patient, money, tokens, food items, etc. may be tried, and automated apparatus for such extrinsic reinforcers may be necessary. Social reinforcement, as was employed by the psychologists, can be highly effective with rehabilitation patients who often have been deprived of this as a result of lengthy confinement, and who have been observed to consider a therapist's attention as highly important.

An effective reinforcer often is one which has been observed to be maintaining undesirable behavior. When the environmental contingencies are altered so that it is given for desired responding this should then increase in frequency while the maladaptive behaviors extinguish, as was the case in the present investigation.

* * * * *

A similar motivational difficulty was treated by Taylor and Persons (1970). A twenty-two-year-old, quadriplegic man had been injured ten months prior to the initiation of the behavior modification program. Although he appeared to be cooperative, his persistence in goal-directed behavior and his sense of responsibility were slight. He participated only minimally in physical therapy and occupational therapy. Despite possessing above average intellectual ability, he had repeated one year of high school and had an inconsistent work history.

From the beginning of his hospitalization, the patient had discussed a desire to attend college as a means of coping with his disability. Although this appeared to be a feasible goal, the staff felt it to be an unrealistic one if he maintained his lack of persistence. It was believed that if a specific program were devised for the patient which would, at least partially, simulate university activities, data would be provided concerning how much intellectual energy he was willing to expend over a period of time. In addition, such a program would give him some practice at working on intellectual tasks, which he had not done in several years.

The activity selected for this program was the amount of time that the patient spent each day in reading behavior. Positive reinforcement was given, in the form of social attention, and withdrawal of this constituted punishment. A bar graph was placed on the patient's wall, and the staff was instructed to comment on his reading and engage in social interaction with him as long as he was maintaining or increasing his reading level. When there was a decrease in reading time from the previous day, the staff's social attention was withheld.

Figure 7-1 presents the data from this study. It shows that before the program's inception the patient read for less than thirty minutes per day. During the first week of the program, he more than doubled his reading time, and during the second week the amount of time he spent reading was more than twice that of the

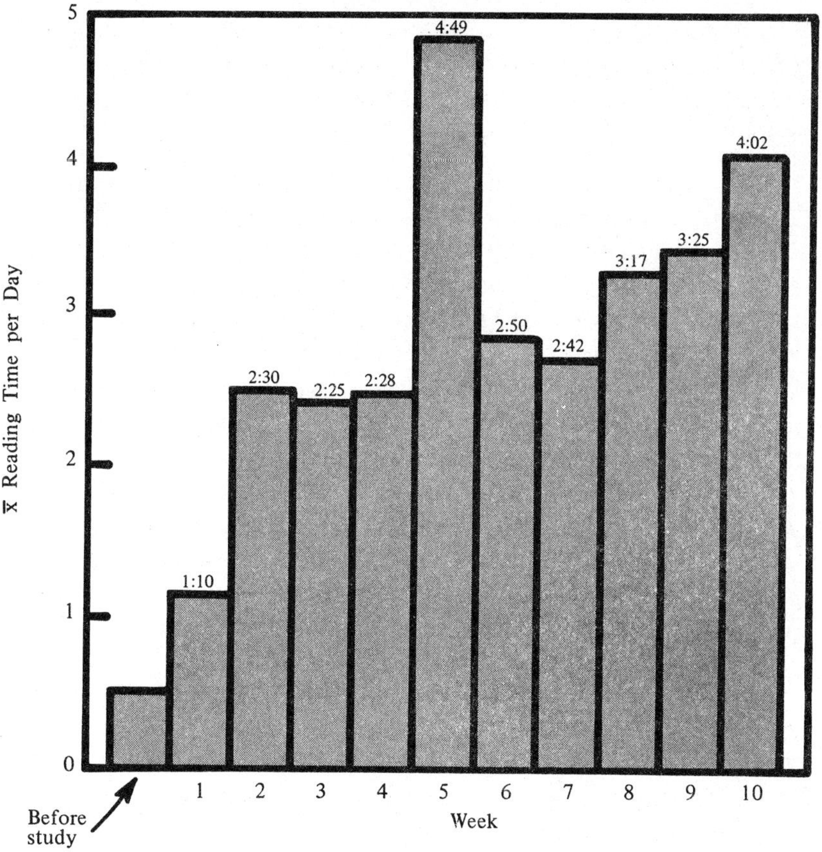

Figure 7-1 Mean number of hours spent reading before and during ten-week study. From Taylor, G. P. and Persons, R. W.: Behavior modification techniques in a physical medicine and rehabilitation center. *J Psychol, 74*:117, 1970.

Reproduced with the permission of the senior author and The Journal Press.

first week. This increase was maintained throughout the ten weeks of the study reaching a peak during the fifth week, and never approximating baseline rate. The patient's mean reading time per day for the experimental period was three hours and nine minutes. This demonstrated that he was capable of increased and sustained goal-directed behavior over a long period of time.

An additional consequence of the program was some generalization to other activities. The patient increased the amount of time he spent typing, and began to correspond actively with various universities with regard to their facilities for disabled students.

A feature of the program which the authors do not discuss was the use of the bar graph, which was displayed publicly. The value of such a device was demonstrated by Fowler, Fordyce and Berni (1969), and by Fordyce, Sand, Trieschmann and Fowler in 1971 (see Chapter Three), and it is possible that the public display of this patient's achievements was highly reinforcing for him. It is also possible that the recorded increases shown on the graph became a conditioned stimulus since they were associated with the reinforcer of social attention.

This investigation again points out the significance of attention and social interaction as reinforcers. It illustrates that hospital personnel must be aware of the effects that even their casual greetings and "small talk" have on patients' behaviors, and that they can and should use this to positive advantage.

The fact that the patient's motivation on one task generalized to other behaviors is important to note. This is a frequently observed phenomenon in rehabilitation. Once a patient who previously appeared to lack motivation finds that he can succeed in a specific area of endeavor, he often becomes motivated to achieve goals in other activities. This may be due to a restoration of his self-concept, increased confidence, or other variables, but the key aspect for the behavioral scientist to be aware of is that engaging successfully in one behavior can lead to engaging in other behaviors. Thus, to motivate a patient, what may be needed is to discover a task on which the patient can be conditioned to respond and then generalization of this responding may occur to other spheres of activity and function.

ATTENDING THERAPY CLASSES

Many disabled patients equate physical therapy with rehabilitation, and have ambulation as their single goal, believing that all they need to do is learn to walk again and that other therapies are unnecessary. This has been found repeatedly to be true, even of patients who require speech therapy and occupational therapy to regain lost functions. As a result of this attitude, patients often attend their physical therapy classes regularly, but do not report for their other prescribed therapy sessions. There then is a tendency for them to be labelled "unmotivated" by the thearpists whose classes they do not attend, and by the physician whose prescription includes a more intensive rehabilitation program.

This was true of two patients whose motivation problems were dealt with effectively by Ince (1969). He utilized the Premack principle (see Premack, 1959, 1962, 1965). Summarized briefly, it holds that of any two responses, the more probable response will reinforce the less probable one. That is, if an organism is in a situation where there are two responses which can be made, an observer could record the relative frequencies with which these responses were made. Then that response which was performed more frequently could be employed as a reinforcer to increase the frequency of occurrence of the other response if it were made contingent upon it.

A sixty-eight-year-old man had suffered a stroke approximately five months before being seen by the psychologist. He had a left hemiparesis and a mild dysarthria, and had been on a rehabilitation program for three months. The program consisted of daily physical therapy (PT), and daily speech therapy (ST). However, the patient only attended PT, stating that once he were able to ambulate independently his "troubles" would be over, and that somehow his speech would return to normal. The speech therapist, on the other hand, reported that he could regain much of his former speech function only if he were to receive therapy on a daily basis.

The investigator made the initial assumption, based upon the patient's observed behavior and verbal remarks, that PT constituted a reinforcing situation for him. Therefore, PT could be employed effectively by making it contingent upon attendance in ST.

The patient's physical therapist was contacted, and the rationale of the Premackian model was explained to him. He was requested not to admit the patient for PT unless he received a call first from the patient's speech therapist informing him that the patient had attended ST earlier in the day. The model also was explained to the speech therapist, who agreed to call the physical therapist daily and inform him as to whether or not the patient had attended his scheduled session with her. The patient was told that he needed a complete rehabilitation program, as prescribed by his physician, if he was to improve in function, and that he was to begin attending all of his therapy classes immediately.

Within three days following the introduction of the contingency system the patient began attending ST on a regular basis. Upon his discharge from the hospital several months later he was still doing so. His attendance in ST had increased from zero to 100 percent of prescribed time, while he maintained his participation in PT at the same level.

* * * * *

The paradigm was extended to include more than two behaviors with a sixty-eight-year-old woman who had sustained a CVA with resultant right hemiplegia, severe expressive and moderate receptive aphasia, and severe apraxia. She was seen by the investigator four months after her admission to a rehabilitation center.

A program of daily therapy classes had been prescribed for her, including PT, occupational therapy (OT) and ST. She refused to attend either OT or ST with any regularity, but attended her PT sessions faithfully.

The patient was told that only participation in a full therapeutic program would be of maximum benefit to her, and that she must make an effort to attend all of her classes. This was repeated to her several times, because of her receptive impairment, until it was certain that she understood what was expected of her.

Her therapy schedule was rearranged so that classes occurred daily in the order of the frequency of her attendance. Thus, OT, which the patient attended only 10 percent of the time, was made the first class of the day. Since she attended ST 25 percent of the prescribed time, this was made her second class. She attended PT 100 percent of her scheduled time, and therefore this was designated as her third, and last class of the day.

The motivation model and its rationale were explained to all of the involved staff members. The occupational therapist was instructed to inform the speech therapist of the patient's attendance, and the speech therapist, in turn, was told to notify the physical therapist. If the occupational therapist reported to the speech therapist that the patient did not attend OT, the speech therapist would not admit her for ST, and made a telephone call to the physical therapist, who would not permit the patient to engage in PT. Thus, a chain was set up whereby the patient either attended all of her therapy classes or could attend none of them. Since her frequency of attendance at PT was so high, it was anticipated that the withdrawal of this reinforcer would act as punishment and would result in increased attendance at all other therapy classes.

The patient initially objected to her revised schedule of classes, and requested that PT be made the first class of the day. When this was not forthcoming, she began to attend her other therapies. Within three days she was attending OT and ST with the same frequency, i.e. 60 percent of the prescribed time. Two days later, this had increased to 80 percent, and after three more days she was attending all of her classes 100 percent of prescribed time. It required a total of only eight days to place this patient on a full rehabilitation program.

The technique employed by Ince in this study required the cooperation of other rehabilitation team members. One therapist initially expressed the feeling that it was "wrong" to deny a patient rehabilitation services even for only a brief period of time. Another stated that she was too busy with other patients to "keep tabs" on one "special" patient. These objections were met with by pointing out that if brief deprivation of one service resulted in the patient's eventually receiving all of the necessary services, then it was preferable to having the patient benefit from only one therapy to the neglect of other important areas, and that all the program required, in addition to the therapist's usual daily work, was to answer one telephone call and/or to make one call, taking approximately one minute per day.

An important point to be made about the procedure concerns the selection of a reinforcer. Often, it is not known what has been reinforcing for a patient in his past history. Much time and effort can be expended in trying to determine an adequate reinforcer for a particular individual. However, this is not necessary when a Premackian model is employed. Over a given time period such as one week, the psychologist or another staff member can observe the patient in his daily activities on his ward or floor, in the hospital corridors, in the canteen, in therapy classes, and wherever the patient spends his time. Frequency samples of each behavior he engages in can be obtained and the behaviors then can be ranked hierarchically, from those he engaged in least to those he engaged in most often. Once this hierarchy is constructed, any behavior can be used to reinforce a behavior which ranks lower on the list; there is no need for trial-and-error experimentation.

This paradigm can be used not only between therapy classes, but within a single therapy situation. For the patient who dislikes manual stretching of contracted extremities and will not permit it to be done, but who enjoys weaving on a loom, weaving can be made contingent upon stretching exercises. The patient who wants to work with a Language Master®, but will not cooperate in performing oral and facial exercises, can be permitted the former only after the latter have been completed. This method appears to provide rehabilitation therapists with a reliable and effective technique for motivating the problem patient.

USING AN EXTREMITY

Friedlander (1973) employed the PLAYTEST system (see Chapter Four) with some unique motivation problems.

A cerebral palsied child had an upper extremity amputated as a result of severe burns. Her response to the amputation was to keep the stump clenched tightly against her body and not use it at all. She also was afraid of losing her balance, and tended to sit in a chair very rigidly.

The child was seated in front of a PLAYTEST console with disc inserts. Plastic cups were affixed onto the two center discs, and the child was required to touch these with her stump in order to activate the switches and receive musical reinforcement. Gradually, she was moved further and further away from the console, and to her own surprise and pleasure she found herself actually moving the stump freely away from her body and becoming much more relaxed in her general body movement. She then was able to be fitted with a prosthesis which she used successfully.

* * * * *

A similar procedure was employed with a seventeen-year-old, cerebral palsied boy who had left-sided spastic hemiplegia, and who never had used his involved arm in any functional manner.

A stick was propped into his hand and under his arm so that he was able to operate the disc modules to receive music as a reinforcer. Then, marks were placed at intervals along the floor in front of the console, and the boy was required to stand progressively further back, necessitating that he reach out with his hand and use the extremity in a coordinated way so as to receive reinforcement.

Although, at first, his time on task was very low, it improved dramatically across test sessions, while his percentage of correct responses always was high. For the first time in his life, he began using his involved extremity functionally.

A FINAL WORD ON MOTIVATION

When a rehabilitation patient does not attend therapy classes, or attends but works half-heartedly, he usually is considered by the staff to be unmotivated. The question then asked is, Why is he not motivated? This is not the appropriate question to pose. What should be asked instead is, what is motivating him not to attend classes and/or to engage in behaviors other than the prescribed therapeutic activities? What are the environmental contingencies which are controlling his behavior?

The term *motivation* really means reinforcement. When we speak about a patient being motivated to perform an activity, we are in fact saying that he is being reinforced for doing so. An experimental analysis must be made of the situation to determine what the reinforcers in the patient's environment are that maintain behaviors which are incompatible with the desired behaviors. It also is possible that the therapy situations themselves have aversive properties for the patient. If so, this must be discovered and dealt with. Once the reinforcement contingencies which are maintaining the undesirable behavior, e.g. not attending therapy, are known, the job becomes one of reversing these contingencies so as to make therapy reinforcing, and other incompatible activities nonreinforcing.

There is no such thing as an unmotivated patient. Every patient is motivated for something. A behavioral analysis can indicate what is reinforcing for the patient in question, and these reinforcers then can be made contingent upon desired responding.

REFERENCES

Friedlander, B. Z.: Physical rehabilitation: applications of research in learning and conditioning. Paper presented at the Conference on Research Utilization for the Rehabilitation of the Disabled Disadvantaged. New York, 1973.

Ince, L. P.: A behavioral approach to motivation in rehabilitation. *Psychol Rec, 19*:105, 1969.

Ince, L. P.: *The Rehabilitation Medicine Services*. Springfield, Thomas, 1974.

Meyerson, L., Kerr, Nancy and Michael, J.: Behavior modification in rehabilitation. In Bijou, S. W. and Baer, D. M. (Eds): *Child Development: Readings in Experimental Analysis*. New York, Appleton-Century-Crofts, 1967.

Premack, D.: Toward empirical behavior laws: I. Positive reinforcement. *Psychol Rev, 66*:219, 1959.

Premack, D.: Reversibility of the reinforcement relation. *Science, 136*:255, 1962.

Premack, D.: Reinforcement theory. In Levine, D. (Ed.): *Nebraska Symposium on Motivation*. Lincoln, Univ. Nebraska Press, 1965.

Taylor, G. P. and Persons, R. W.: Behavior modification techniques in a physical medicine and rehabilitation center. *J Psychol, 74*:117, 1970.

Chapter Eight

DISRUPTIVE BEHAVIORS

WHILE DISRUPTIVE PATIENT behaviors do occur in an acute medical setting, they are observed more frequently in a rehabilitation institution. There are several reasons for this. As pointed out earlier, rehabilitation patients are confined to relatively close quarters for comparatively long periods of time. The hospital population also is fairly representative of a cross section of society. Thus, the kinds of behavior problems encountered in a community are met with in the institutional setting, which tends to become a "mini-community" of its own.

In addition, rehabilitation patients exhibit many of the problems which result directly from the fact that they are disabled or seriously ill. Anger, hostility, acting out, complaining, negativism, etc. are consequences of the anxieties, frustrations and depressions felt by the patients who no longer can function as they did prior to the onset of their disorder. Impulsive behaviors, noisiness, quarreling, and the like can stem from brain injuries which produce such reactions or remove the cortical inhibitions to responding in these ways.

Furthermore, although many undesirable behaviors are the direct result of the physical handicaps, others may have existed prior to a patient's disability and have been exacerbated by it.

For these reasons, the psychologist and the other rehabilitation team members often have a difficult time in the area of patient management. A patient's maladaptive behavior can interfere not only with his own rehabilitation progress, but with that of others as well, and can have a seriously disrupting influence on his floor or ward, or in therapy areas. Disruptive behaviors, therefore, must be dealt with, and sometimes very swiftly.

This chapter presents some of the techniques which behavioral scientists employ in dealing with problems of this nature.

COMPLAINING

Taylor and Persons (1970) used social reinforcement in treating two cases of complaining behavior.

A fifty-four-year-old housewife with multiple sclerosis was admitted to a rehabilitation center, and during her first week of hospitalization was such a bitter and chronic complainer that both the staff and other patients found her to be disturbing and disruptive. She became an outcast among the patients, and the quality of care that she was receiving from the staff progressively deteriorated. After one week she returned home for three weeks, and then reentered the hospital. During the three-week hiatus it was decided by the staff to utilize behavior modification techniques to reduce the ward management problems presented by the patient, and to prevent her from disturbing those around her.

Social attention was selected as the reinforcer. It was made contingent upon lack of complaining. The first step of the modification program was the sensitization of the patient to the frequency of her complaints. She was given a wrist counter to wear daily, and each time she complained she was to depress the recording button on the counter. When she went to bed, the night nurse recorded the total that was registered on the counter, and reset it to zero. Wrist counters also were worn by the patient's physical therapist and occupational therapist, and they recorded the number of times that the patient complained during her sessions with them.

The second procedure involved social interaction with the patient when she did not complain. When she offered complaints, this was kept to a minimum. The hospital staff was friendly, and engaged the patient in conversation as long as she maintained her noncomplaining behavior, but did not do this when she complained.

The results of the behavior modification program are presented in Figure 8-1. It is obvious that during the first four days the patient's own count of the number of times she complained differed significantly from the frequencies arrived at by her therapists. As the program continued and she became more aware of the chronicity of her behavior, her self-reports agreed more and more with the reports of the therapists.

There was a dramatic decrease in the number of complaints

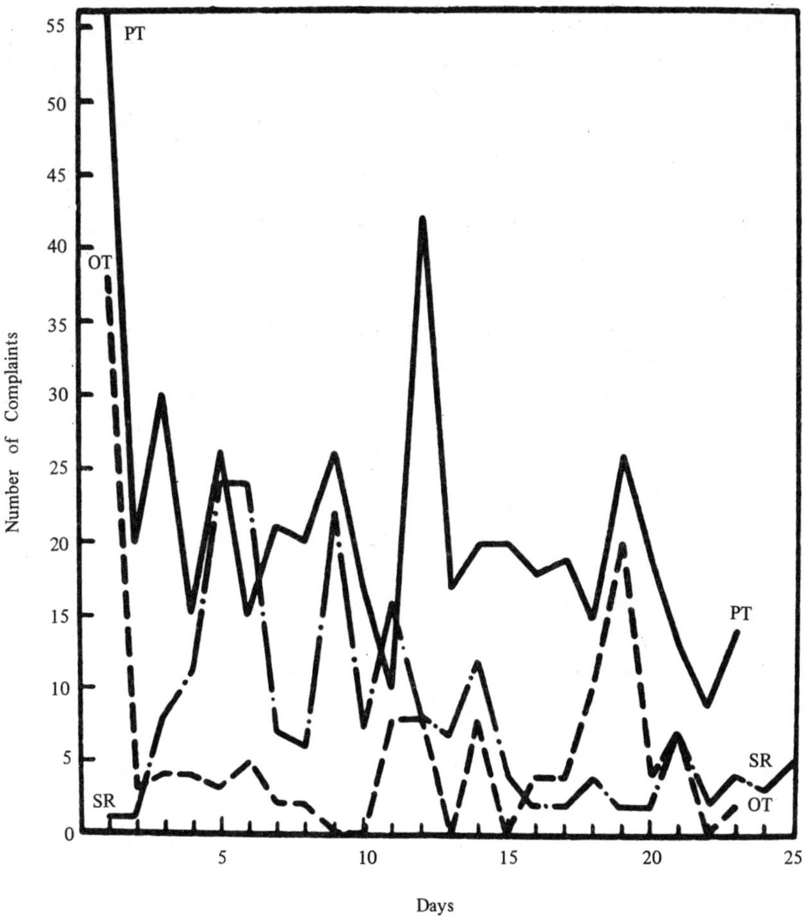

Figure 8-1 Physical therapists (PT), occupational therapists (OT) and patient's self-report (SR) of daily complaining behavior. From Taylor, G. P. and Persons, R. W.: Behavior modification techniques in a physical medicine and rehabilitation center. *J Psychol, 74*:117, 1970.

Reproduced with the permission of the senior author and The Journal Press.

recorded by both the physical therapist and the occupational therapist after only one day of the reinforcement contingency arrangement. With few exceptions, the rate of the patient's complaints continued to decrease during the study. Observation of the patient in the hospital, and comments made by the staff, also revealed a marked reduction of the complaining behavior. Her problems at the rehabilitation center simultaneously declined, and the other patients became much more receptive to her.

* * * * *

The second case was that of a thirty-seven-year-old man with quadriparesis resulting from an automobile accident. During the first week of his hospitalization, he emitted psychotic verbalizations and engaged in many dependency-type behaviors. He complained continually about various psychiatric problems, and besieged numerous staff members for psychotherapy. Therapy was considered contraindicated by the staff for several reasons, and behavior modification was chosen as the treatment of choice.

Attention was withheld from the patient whenever he talked about his psychiatric complaints. Concurrently, attention was given for talking about other topics, particularly progress in physical or occupational therapy. This system of punishment and reinforcement was in effect for three months.

The behavior modification procedures resulted in a highly significant reduction of complaining. Concomitantly, they increased the patient's independence, cooperativeness, likeability, and general adjustment and adaptation to the rehabilitation program.

Once again, the importance of staff attention to a patient is recognized, as this reinforcer was employed successfully with both patients. Also, as has been found by other investigators, generalization occurred from improvement in the target behavior to other areas of responding.

This study provides a clear example of the importance of staff cooperation in achieving a desired goal. In rehabilitation, the other disciplines expect the psychologist to use his armamentarium of skills and techniques to alleviate any difficulties which arise with a patient. Very often he is able to accomplish this without assistance from others. However, there are many times when he cannot handle the task alone, either because he cannot maintain the necessary observation and control as the patient traverses the numerous areas of the hospital, or because other staff members are, albeit unknowingly, responding to the patient in ways that contradict what the psychologist is attempting to accomplish. Therefore, there are many instances in which the psychologist must rely upon the cooperation of other professionals. The concept of rehabilitation as a team effort extends to the behavior management sphere.

NEGATIVISM

As is true of the physical therapist and the occupational therapist, the speech clinician also encounters behaviors which interfere with therapeutic processes.

The majority of the studies which are described in this chapter deal with the extinction of undesirable behavior through punishment techniques, or by reinforcement of incompatible behaviors. Kushner and Knox (1973), however, employed a different method, one developed by Erickson (1959), known as the "utilization technique," to eliminate the negativistic behavior of a rehabilitation patient.

This method emphasizes gaining control over an undesirable behavior. Instead of ignoring or punishing the behavior, the clinician utilizes it. The patient is encouraged to engage in it, but to do so under the clinician's direction. Once this is accomplished, the clinician channels the direction of responding into a more cooperative activity.

The patient with whom this technique was employed was a twenty-five-year-old man with diffuse brain damage as the consequence of an automobile accident. He had been diagnosed as having trauma, secondary to brain stem contusion. He was referred for speech therapy because of inappropriate verbalizations and inconsistent communication. His other therapists and ward personnel considered him to be uncooperative, and reported that he sat in his wheelchair with his head tilted backward, refusing to participate in rehabilitation activities.

The speech therapist initially attempted to determine the

extent of the patient's communication deficit. However, his uncooperative behavior disrupted the diagnostic sessions so that an evaluation could not be performed. He tilted his head back, stared at the ceiling, and stated that he was unable to look at the test materials as the therapist directed.

In the first session during which the utilization technique was applied, the patient was wheeled to a table which held the test materials. The therapist requested the patient to perform a task, and he responded by claiming that he could not see the materials. The therapist then instructed him to keep his head in the backward-tilted position and stare at the ceiling. The patient then pulled his head forward and performed the required tasks appropriately for the remainder of the session.

At the beginning of the next session, the patient held his head tilted backwards. The therapist responded to this behavior by saying, "I want you to keep your head back and stare at the ceiling." As before, the patient pulled his head forward and maintained it properly while he engaged in the required tasks until the session ended.

During the third session, the patient began resisting the therapist's instructions to tilt his head backward. He told her that he didn't like to be "ordered around," and that he did not want to hold his head back because then he could not see her nor the test materials. He kept his head forward throughout the period, and for the next three sessions as well.

When the therapist saw the patient at the start of the seventh session, he again had his head tilted backward and was staring at the ceiling. This was the result of the secretarial staff praising him for "looking nice" because his head was held properly. The patient's response to the praise was to revert to his previous maladaptive behavior.

The therapist encouraged him to keep his head back, and once again the patient pulled it forward, complaining that he could not see anything in that position. He continued to hold his head appropriately, and perform the necessary tasks until the evaluation was completed, the findings of which revealed that therapy was not indicated.

The results of the utilization technique with this patient indicated that by encouraging him to resist, it was possible for the therapist to get him to give up his undesirable behavior. Kushner and Knox state that for a problemmatic behavior to persist it must have a marked influence on another person, and the patient must somehow indicate that the behavior he is engaging in is beyond his control. If this is true, the strength of the patient's behavior, in the case just presented, may have been weakened by its utilization because the therapist communicated to him that she was not influenced by him, and that she did not really believe that he could not help what he was doing. Her encouragement of the undesirable behavior placed the patient in a situation where, when he cooperated he was following the therapist's instructions, and when he did not cooperate he was behaving as the therapist wanted. His behavior thus became ineffective in controlling his environment.

Another approach, which a different therapist might have attempted with this patient, would have been to hold or suspend the test materials above his head in such a way that when his head was tilted backward he could see and respond to them. It might have been thought that this would have the effect of not permitting his behavior to enable him to avoid the tasks. However, this actually would have been reinforcing the patient's undesirable response, since his behavior would then be controlling that of the therapist and the evaluation procedures. By not doing this, the patient did not gain control over the situation and his behavior had no positive consequences for him.

BELLIGERENCE

Hostility and aggression are among the most undesirable behaviors which a rehabilitation patient can emit. They present particular difficulties for the staff since, by their nature, they are highly disruptive and prevent progress in therapy, and also because they usually must be dealt with promptly and cannot be ignored.

Hollon (1973) successfully managed a problem of this type. A twenty-two-year-old woman had suffered severe cerebral contusion and a decompressed skull fracture in an automobile accident.

While she exhibited some regression and disorientation, it was felt by the rehabilitation staff that she had considerable potential for return of motoric, speech and intellectual functions. After two weeks on the rehabilitation program, however she became extremely belligerent and disruptive. She persistently howled for long periods of time. Whenever anyone attempted to learn the reasons for her behavior, or attempted to stop it, she tried to hit and scratch the person while emitting a torrent of profanity. Therapy became an impossible chore, and the patient's relationships with her nurses had deteriorated into a constant battle. In order to eliminate these behaviors which, if continued, would necessitate transfer of the patient to a custodial institution, a behavior modification approach was used.

Observation of the situation revealed that it was the undesirable responses, i.e. hitting, scratching, cursing and howling, which received the greatest amount of attention and staff time. The nurses and the therapists, in their efforts to eliminate the belligerent behavior, were instead reinforcing it. Therefore, they were instructed to exert only enough force to prevent the patient from hitting and scratching. Otherwise, they were to ignore her disruptive behavior completely.

It had been noted that at times the patient assumed an alert attitude when she asked simple questions about matters such as visitors or when meals were going to be served. This behavior presented no difficulties for the staff, and it typically was ignored. Since, on the other hand, it did inhibit the problemmatic behaviors, the staff was instructed to encourage it. When the patient was alert and questioning, they were to reinforce her with special attention. The reinforcer consisted of clasping both of her hands firmly, and speaking to her in a reassuring manner for several minutes.

The psychologist worked with the patient for one hour each morning, and one hour in the afternoon. She encouraged the patient to assume the alert demeanor, and to ask questions by saying to her, "Talk to me. Tell me what is troubling you," and the like. When the patient responded with conversation, or by asking questions, the psychologist reinforced her by replying, "That's fine. It's good for you to talk to me," and similar statements. She also answered questions posed by the patient.

This general approach was used by other staff members during the day. The patient's mother also was instructed in the behavior modification techniques, and she participated in the program during her visits to the hospital and when the patient was at home.

Within one week after the introduction of the behavioral procedures the patient no longer howled. Hitting, scratching and cursing had markedly been reduced, and the patient's capacity to carry on a conversation without belligerence had increased. Over the next two weeks, her hitting, scratching, and use of profanity were eliminated entirely except for occasional outbursts. She also engaged more frequently in conversations with the staff.

The next major step consisted of reinforcing the patient only when her desirable behavior, i.e. alertness, questioning, engaging in dialogue, was accompanied by her assistance with making her bed or with preparing her bath. Following this, she was reinforced for a behavioral chain, consisting of alertness, conversing, carrying out self-help activities, and going to and participating in therapy classes. Her occasional outbursts were ignored.

Over a five-week period, her behavior had reached the point where she was able to participate fully in her rehabilitation therapies and cooperate maximally in her self-care.

At first, the hospital staff had considered the patient's behavior to be unmanageable. It was extremely difficult to ignore, and personnel felt that they had the burden of dealing with it in some way. The behavior modification approach changed their role to that of observers of the patient's behavior in order to identify potentially constructive patterns. They could use their skills and ingenuity then to get the patient to respond in the ways which they themselves had designated as desirable. Thus, not only was a previously unmanageable patient made accessable to therapy, but patient-staff relations were improved through appropriate interactions.

This study demonstrates the necessity of ordering priorities in dealing with problems such as those presented by this patient. The primary goal was a reduction of the aggressive and disruptive behaviors. This was of immediate concern and had to be treated first. Since the patient also demonstrated an alert, questioning attitude at times, it was possible to reinforce this simultaneously, but in any case the belligerent responses required first consideration. Once these were brought under control, it became possible to proceed gradually with the reinforcement of desirable responses. Had the psychologist ordered the priorities differently, it is questionable if the results would have been as satisfactory.

* * * * *

A similar problem was treated in a different manner by Sand, Trieschmann, Fordyce and Fowler (1970). A four-and-one-half-year-old boy became brain damaged as a result of being thrown from a horse. He was able to ambulate with a wheeled walkerette, and could use a few words following an initial rehabilitation effort six months postinjury. At the age of seven years, he was readmitted to a rehabilitation hospital for further therapy because he had made little additional progress in ambulation and self-care since his first hospitalization.

However, frequent temper tantrums became a significant problem. The child's tantrums were characterized by spitting at, kicking, hitting and biting nearby therapy staff members, and by loud screaming. These occurred as often as six times per day during the first ten days of his hospital stay. The tantrums occurred most frequently when he was asked to do something which was mildly uncomfortable, such as physical therapy exercises, or when he was requested to try a new activity, e.g. self-feeding. His disruptive behaviors resulted in most of his therapy sessions being terminated early, sometimes after only ten minutes of treatment. While the child understood his need for rehabilitation, and appeared to like his therapists, his refusal to cooperate and his tantrums seriously were hindering all therapeutic efforts.

In determining the best methods for dealing with the patient's maladaptive behaviors, the investigators observed that the attention he was receiving for these behaviors appeared to be maintaining their frequency. In addition, they felt that signs of progress would not be as clear or as meaningful to a child as they were for adults. Therefore, tangible, extrinsic reinforcers were utilized, contingent upon proper behavior.

The nurses and the therapists were instructed to put the child in his room for fifteen minutes as soon as he began a tantrum, and to do this in a casual, matter-of-fact manner. This gave him little opportunity to act out in their presence, and they in turn had little opportunity to pay attention to the tantrum behaviors. After each of these time-out periods, a staff member would enter his room pleasantly and take him back to the treatment area.

In order to improve compliance with requests, the nurses and the rehabilitation therapists gave the child tokens when he did as he was instructed, or when he worked on new or difficult tasks. At the end of each day, these tokens could be exchanged for small toys, extra juice, candy, a picnic lunch with a nurse outside the hospital, or other tangible rewards.

During the fifth week, an eight-day period was introduced, during which neither tokens nor time-out periods were used, but praise was given for good performance. Observations were made during this time to determine the effects of this on his behavior. After eight days, time-out was reinstated for disruptive behaviors, and tokens were delivered again for cooperation in therapy.

Figure 8-2 shows the effects of the program on the child's behavior in physical therapy, and Figure 8-3 presents the data for occupational therapy. *Period A* in both figures represents the pretreatment period. Refusal to do as he was asked and verbal tantrums were estimated by his therapists as occurring in every physical therapy session, while 80 percent of the sessions were characterized by physical tantrums. The occupational therapists estimated verbal tantrums to occur nearly 100 percent of the time, refusals to occur approximately 75 percent of the time, and physical tantrums happening about 45 percent of therapy time.

The treatment plan was begun in *Period B,* and both figures indicate a marked decline of all disruptive behaviors. When the contingencies were withdrawn during *Period C,* there was a significant increase in disruptive behaviors during physical therapy, but not in occuaptional therapy. This was assumed to happen because in occupational therapy the patient's behaviors had come under the control of social cues such as attention, approval, and intrinsic reinforcement.

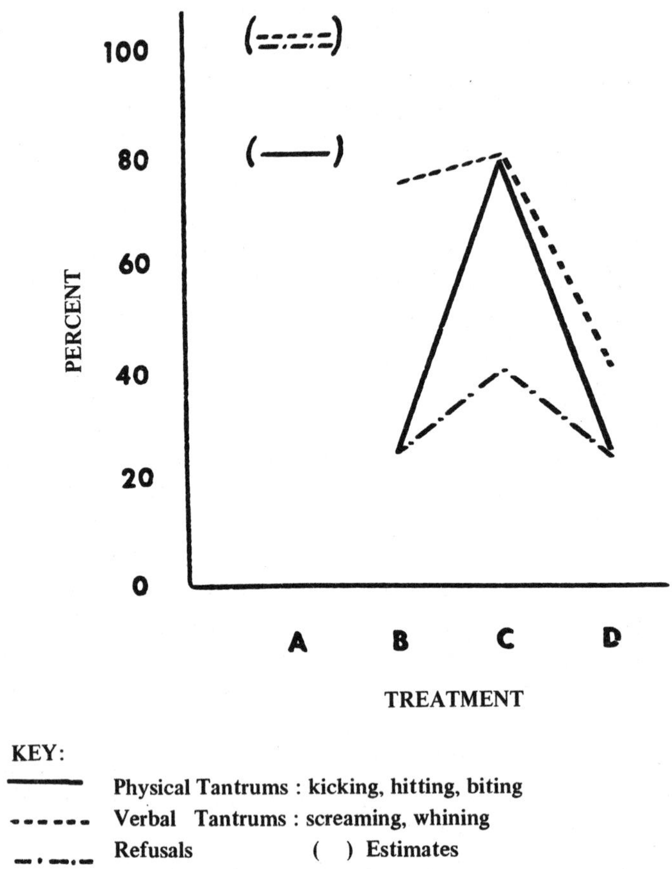

Figure 8-2 Occurrence of problem behaviors in physical therapy. From Sand, Patricia L., Trieschmann, Roberta B., Fordyce, W. E. and Fowler, R. S.: Behavior modification in the medical rehabilitation setting: Rationale and some applications. *Rehab Res Pract Rev, 1*:11, 1970.

Reproduced with the permission of the senior author and the *Rehabilitation Research and Practice Review,* Arkansas Rehabilitation Research and Training Center.

Based upon this finding, the token program was discontinued in occupational therapy, hence no data are presented for *Period D* in Figure 8.3. When the program was resumed in physical therapy

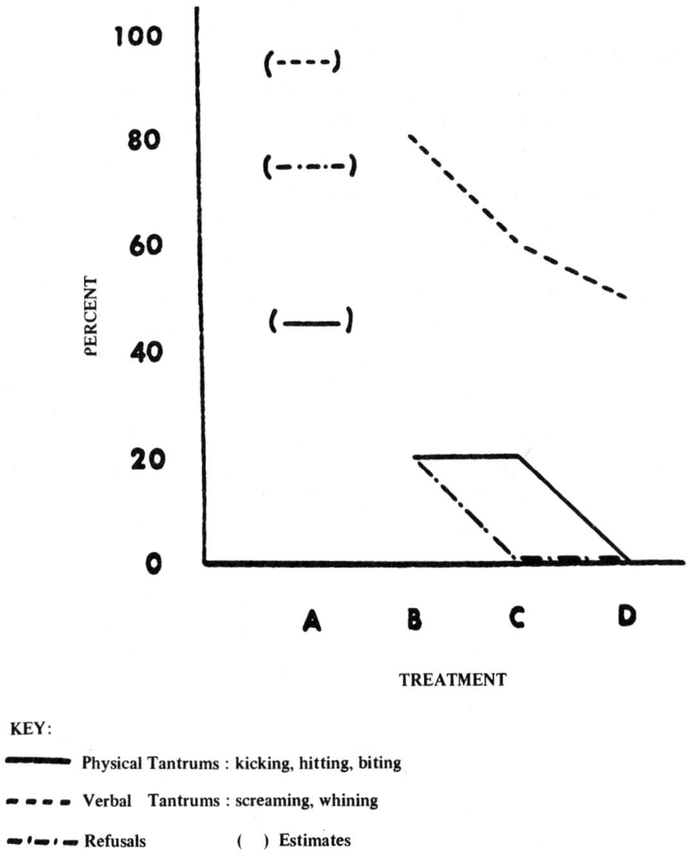

Figure 8-3 Occurrence of problem behaviors in occupational therapy. From Sand, Patricia L., Trieschmann, Roberta B., Fordyce, W. E. and Fowler, R. S.: Behavior modification in the medical rehabilitation setting: Rationale and some applications. *Rehab Res Pract Rev, 1*:11, 1970.

Reproduced with the permission of the senior author and the *Rehabilitation Research and Practice Review,* Arkansas Rehabilitation Research and Training Center.

(*Period D*), problem behaviors again significantly declined.

When the child's hospitalization had come to an end, he had made excellent progress in independent ambulation and self-feeding. In addition, he was a cheerful and well-behaved child with whom the staff enjoyed spending their free time.

A point worth mentioning about this study is the decision to use tangible reinforcers rather than attention or verbal praise, which frequently have been employed, or intrinsic reinforcers, such as a "good feeling" as a result of making progress in therapy. It is to be expected that a child would not be as aware of gains made in therapy, especially slight ones, as would an adult. Thus, intrinsic feelings of satisfaction would either not be present, or would not be of sufficient strength to modify a behavior problem. It also is to be anticipated that the goals determined by the professional staff would not precisely be those of a child. However, receiving a toy or a piece of candy, or having a picnic, are clear, meaningful rewards and signs of doing well.

This is true not only of children but with certain adults as well, particularly those who have sustained some form of brain injury where their ability to reason abstractly is impaired. Many patients do not understand the need for, or relevance of certain activities in their recovery process, even when the reasons for engaging in them have been explained by their therapists. Thus, there is little intrinsic motivation for them to perform these tasks well. Furthermore, attention and praise may not have the same meaning or importance for the patient as the therapist expects, and thus, are not powerful reinforcers. In such cases, it is wise to substitute more concrete reinforcers, such as cigarettes or coffee, for example. In the determination of an appropriate reinforcer, one must always consider the patient for whom it is intended.

Multiple Problems

Many rehabilitation patients present more than one maladaptive behavior in need of treatment. Sometimes, several procedures are required to modify them, with a different technique being applied to each one. In other instances, a single procedure can be employed effectively with all of the difficulties. The latter is more typically the case, since the contingencies controlling one behavior usually are maintaining similar control over the others, and what is reinforcing or punishing for a patient in one situation will also be reinforcing or punishing for him in another. It usually is preferable to employ one set of techniques since this simplifies the methodology and presents fewer problems to the various staff members who may have to become involved in the behavior modification program. Both of the studies described in this section are examples of the single method approach.

Osborne (1970) treated the numerous behavioral difficulties presented by a fifteen-year-old girl with bilateral hearing loss and athetosis of the upper extremities. Despite possessing an IQ within the Dull-Normal range, she was doing little academic work. She also was careless with regard to her personal hygiene and did not get along well with her peers. In addition, she often was late for classes and meals, did not keep her bed area neat and clean, and exhibited such undesirable behaviors as using profanity, losing her temper, and responding negatively to reasonable requests made by the staff. The investigation was conducted in a residential school for the deaf, where her behavior problems had progressed to the point where discharge was being considered.

The psychologist decided to reinforce the girl with activities which she desired, contingent upon proper conduct. She would have to earn points by behaving appropriately, and these points then could be exchanged for the "payoff" activities.

The goal of the experiment was the reduction of undesirable responses and the increase of correct behaviors. Table 8-I lists the responses in the problem areas and the number of points which could be earned for correct behaviors in each response subclass.

All of the responses in the positive response class could occur only under physically limited circumstances. Responses which were emitted under a wrong set of circumstances were not reinforced. Thus, doing homework for classes received reinforcement, but doing extra, unrequired homework did not. These positive responses were termed *controlled operants.* The responses in the negative class were labelled *free operants,* meaning that there was no limit to the number of them which would receive punishment.

Response Class	*Response-Subclass*	*Points Available*	*Total Points Possible*
	Positive Responses		
Being on time	a.) to meals	3 daily	15
	b.) to class	5 daily	25
	c.) to gym	1 Mon. & Tues.	2
		Week Total	42
Personal care	a.) teeth brushed	3 daily	15
	b.) hair combed	3 daily	15
	c.) face washed	3 daily	15
		Week Total	45
Cleanliness	a.) bed made	5 daily	25
	b.) clothes put away	5 daily	25
	c.) room cleaned	50 once/week	50
	d.) clothes washed	50 once/week	50
	e.) clothes ironed	50 once/week	50
		Week Total	200
Dorm duty*		10 daily	50
		Week Total	50
Academic work	a.) homework	50 each academic class, 3 classes 5 days/week	750
	b.) classwork	50 each class, 5 classes, 5 days/ week	1250
		Week Total	2000
		Grand Total	2337
	Negative Responses		
Deportment	a.) swearing	−50 each instance	
	b.) losing temper	−50 each instance	
	c.) refusal of reasonable requests	−50 each instance	
		Week Total	Unlimited

*This activity was variable consisting of approximately ten minutes of cleaning work in the dorm besides S's room.

Table 8-I Response classes and subclasses with the number of points available for each response. From Osborne, J. G.: Behavior modification with a deaf student: A case study. *Psychol Asp Disabil, 17*:71, 1970.

Reproduced with the permission of the author and *Rehabilitation Psychology* (formerly *Psychological Aspects of Disability*).

Each response to be modified was objectively defined. For example, *Being on time to meals* was defined as being seated at the correct table in the cafeteria when the meal began. *Personal hygiene* and *Cleanliness* were observed by dormitory personnel, or if the actual activity could not be observed, it was inferred from such characteristics as combed hair, clean face, etc., or made bed, clothes neatly put away, and the like. *Losing temper* was defined as any excessive response, verbal or motor, that was considered by the staff as deserving of punishment. Punishment also was given for profanity, and for refusing to follow instructions or responding negatively to reasonable staff requests. The girl's teachers assigned homework daily, each teacher giving approximately one hour of homework per hour of class time.

Point values for each response subclass were determined following observation. Since *Academic work* and *Deportment* were considered to be the classes in which behavioral changes were most needed, they were assigned the most points.

The reinforcers were selected and hierarchically ordered on the basis of interviews with the staff and observations of the girl. These are presented in Table 8-II.

Activity	*Cost*
Go home for the weekend	2200
Parents visit on the weekend	2000
Go to shopping center	400
Movie downtown	400
Movie at school	400
Buy candy	200
Watch T.V. each evening	75

Table 8-II Payoff activities available to the subject each Friday with their individual point cost. From Osborne, J. G.: Behavior modification with a deaf student: A case study. *Psychol Asp Disabil, 17*:71, 1970.

Reproduced with the permission of the author and *Rehabilitation Psychology* (formerly *Psychological Aspects of Disability*).

Seven electrically operated counters were placed in the girl's room. Six were labelled with the response classes of the study: five for the positive behaviors and one for the negative behaviors. Negative points were subtracted from the total of positive points and the remainder was recorded on the seventh counter.

Two weeks prior to initiating the point system, the critical responses were observed and recorded by the staff. During this baseline period the girl was unaware that her behavior was being measured.

At the beginning of the third week, the girl was shown the counters and informed that certain behaviors would earn her points, while others would lose points for her. She was told that each Friday she would be able to exchange the points she had earned during the week for desired activities. The response subclasses and the "payoff" activities were explained to her, and she was told that the experimenter would total her point earnings each day after school. She always was informed as to what her points were for, e.g. making her bed, getting to class on time, and so on.

Each Friday, the girl was given the opportunity to select as many of the "payoff" activities as her point total for the week permitted. She was requested to spend all of her points so that the counters could be reset to zero for the following week.

The study was conducted over a ten-week period. The sixth and seventh weeks were used as control conditions. Following each of these weeks the girl was permitted to choose a "payoff" activity without any required behavioral contingency. No points were recorded on the counters during these weeks, but observation and recording of her behavior was maintained. If the point system was controlling her behavior, it would be expected that positive responses would decrease, while negative ones increased, during the control weeks.

Figure 8-4 illustrates the weekly changes in the two response classes initially designated as requiring the greatest modification. The data for *Academic work* are presented in the upper portion of the figure, and the data for *Deportment* can be seen in the lower portion.

It is clear that far more academic work was completed during the experimental periods, when points were earned, than during the control weeks, when reinforcement was not contingent upon points. It also is obvious that undesirable behaviors decreased when they resulted in a loss of points, and increased when they did not have such a consequence. The differences between baseline measurements and first conditioning periods were highly significant for both classes of responses.

Less dramatic changes were obtained in the other four classes of behavior, but their premodification baseline rates already were

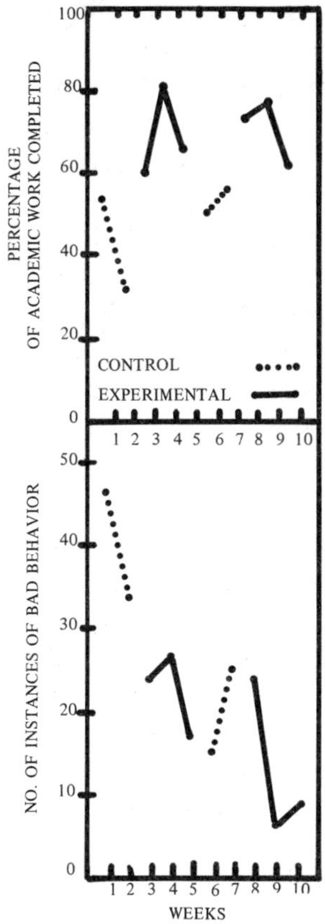

Figure 8-4 Changes in *Academic work* (upper) and *Deportment* (lower) response classes by the week. From Osborne, J. G.: Behavior modification with a deaf student: A case study. *Psychol Asp Disabil, 17*:71, 1970.

Reproduced with the permission of the author and *Rehabilitation Psychology* (formerly *Psychological Aspects of Disability*).

high, contrary to the staff's beliefs, and little experimental change had been expected. During the control weeks, two of the desirable behaviors, *Dorm duty* and *Cleanliness* markedly declined, but they increased again once the contingencies were reinstated.

The use of baseline measurements and a control period makes this study unique among those discussed in this chapter. As pointed out in Chapter Two, these generally are considered crucial, since without premodification measures the effects of a specific procedure cannot adequately be assessed. Nonetheless, many studies are conducted without an initial baseline period. From a scientific standpoint, this is not justifiable. However, from a practical point of view, it often is necessary.

In a rehabilitation setting, the primary objectives pertain to patient care, clinical treatment, and not to scientific research. Thus, for patients who are in need of health care services, it usually is not feasible or possible to withhold delivery of this care until adequate baseline data has been collected. This is true particularly in emergency situations where the health and medical well-being of a patient is the consideration, or when a patient's maladaptive behavior endangers him or others, or prevents him or others from participating in rehabilitation therapies. In these instances, modification of behavior must be carried out as rapidly as possible, sacrificing sound scientific procedure for the necessity of immediate action for change.

In almost all of the studies presented in this and other chapters, where a baseline phase was not employed, the behavioral scientist was consulted after other staff members had observed the patient's behavior for a considerable period of time. Thus, there was baseline data in a sense, even if only in anecdotal form. Nonetheless, when immediacy of action is not required, such casual observations and reports are not adequate substitutes for scientific correctness. This is illustrated by Osborne's investigation, wherein he did use a baseline phase and learned that four of the response classes designated for modification had, in fact, much higher frequencies of occurrence than the opinions of the staff initially had led him to believe.

The interjection of a control period was important since it demonstrated the effectiveness of the point system. Had the girl's responses remained unchanged during these two weeks it would have been obvious that variables other than the experimental ones were controlling her behavior.

A token system also was employed by Hurwitz (1973) in altering the numerous behavior problems exhibited by a twenty-eight-year-old man. As a consequence of head trauma, the patient had suffered a skull fracture and a left subdural hematoma, which produced a right hemiparesis and severe expressive and moderate receptive aphasia. He was ambulatory and had normal use of his left upper extremity and good use of his right arm. He was independent in all activities of daily living.

For three years prior to being placed on a behavior modification program, the patient posed considerable management problems in the chronic care section of the rehabilitation hospital. There were four primary maladaptive behaviors which the program was designed to reduce. These were: frequent fighting with the staff and other patients; frequent alcoholic intoxication; leaving the hospital without a pass; and wearing "street" clothes without permission. (The patient had, on several occasions, simply left the hospital without informing anyone. On one of these occasions he was badly beaten physically by unknown assailants, and in another instance, returned to the hospital severely frost-bitten. As part of the staff's attempts to discourage this behavior, he was not permitted to wear his own clothing and was restricted to wearing hospital garb only.)

The most effective reinforcer for the patient, as determined by the psychologist, was wearing his own clothing. He was a vain man, and his appearance meant a great deal to him. Observations of the patient and interviews with him clearly had shown this to be the most desired reward for him.

In order for him to be able to wear his clothing for one day, he had to exhibit correct behavior for seven consecutive days. Correct behavior was defined as behavior which did not include any of the previously mentioned problem responses, i.e. fighting, drinking alcoholic beverages, leaving the hospital and wearing his own clothing.

A chart, in the form of a calendar, was placed by the patient's bed. At the end of each day of correct behavior, the patient pasted a gummed silver star in the appropriate space on the chart. After seven consecutive silver stars had been pasted onto the chart, he pasted a gold star in the space for the following day, and wore his own clothing during that one day. Thus, one week of correct behavior (Monday through Sunday) resulted in one day of reinforcement (Monday).

The reinforcement was delivered according to a constantly changing schedule which permitted greater reinforcement for greater time periods of good conduct. Thus, for the first two weeks of the program, seven consecutive days of good behavior earned one day of clothing. For the third and fourth weeks, seven days of good behavior resulted in two days of reinforcement. Correct behavior during the fifth and sixth weeks permitted the patient to wear his clothing for three days. This shifting ratio was maintained until by the thirteenth and fourteenth weeks the patient was allowed to wear his clothing for seven days if his behavior had been appropriate during the seven preceding days.

The stars were placed on the chart at the end of each day by the patient. During the first week of the program, the psychologist glued the stars in the appropriate spaces, but from the second week on, the patient was "on his honor" to reinforce himself correctly.

If the patient engaged in any of the undesirable behaviors, he was to paste a red star in the appropriate chart space. When this occurred, he would be told immediately, by the psychologist or a nurse, that he could not wear his clothing the following day, regardless of what the current reinforcement schedule called for, and on the following day he would have to begin a new seven-day period of good behavior to earn reinforcement.

The behavior modification program — rationale, goals and procedures — were explained to the staff of the three nursing shifts on the patient's ward, and the cooperation of the nurses was enlisted. A duplicate of the patient's bedside chart was kept in his medical record at the ward nursing station. Each day, the psychologist pasted a star in this chart so that the nurses could follow the patient's progress, and could compare the psychologist's judgement of the patient's behavior with their own judgements, and with that of the patient. During weekends, the nurses were responsible for maintaining the chart at the nursing station. While the patient had primary responsibility for the accuracy of his bedside chart, the psychologist verified the validity of the patient's self-ratings with his nurses.

The nature and purposes of the program were explained to the patient and he agreed to participate.

The token system was highly successful in eliminating the patient's undesirable behaviors. From the first day of its inception he received a silver star every day for fourteen consecutive weeks. He never exhibited any of the maladaptive behaviors which the study had been designed to treat, and hence, never received a punishing red star. The ratings of the patient's behavior by the psychologist and the nurses correlated nearly perfectly with his self-ratings.

In addition to the immediate and total cessation of all of his previous problemmatic behaviors, the patient began to assume more responsibility for his own daily conduct. He was given weekend passes on several occasions and always returned to the hospital on time and without incident. He became more helpful in assisting other, more disabled patients in the hospital, and generally was considered by all to be a "model" patient.

One year after the termination of the behavior modification program, the patient was maintaining his problem-free and cooperative behavior without a single recurrence of the difficulties which he had presented for three years prior to the study.

This study is an example of what might clinically be termed "errorless" learning. That is, once the program began, the patient never misbehaved. Hurwitz felt that there were two reasons for this. *First,* the psychologist previously had worked closely with the patient, therapeutically, and therefore had established good rapport and credibility with him. The psychologist had been empathetic, accepting and understanding of the patient and his problems, and the patient, in turn, was willing to attempt what the psychologist asked of him. *Second,* although numerous forms of punishment for maladaptive behaviors had been tried by the staff over the years, the patient never before had been deprived of his clothing. As mentioned previously, the patient was a vain man and he felt degraded and embarrassed in hospital garb. He refused to attend physical therapy or speech therapy while so dressed, yet when he was wearing his own clothing he went to his therapy classes regularly. The importance that his clothing had for him was obvious to the psychologist who used it as the key to modifying his behavior.

* * * * *

A criticism that often is levelled at behavior modification by those who are unknowledgeable in its principles and methods is that it is a mechanistic, dehumanizing and authoritarian way of dealing with an individual's problems. As many of the studies discussed in this chapter illustrate, nothing could be further from the truth. Behavior modification techniques are never generically applied, but always are geared specifically to the particular individual in question. His needs, his wants, his goals are the primary consideration. Every patient is viewed as a unique individual, to be treated as such, and specific techniques for specific problems of specific individuals is a cardinal rule.

Furthermore, whenever possible, the nature of the techniques, the rationale behind their use, and the goals and purposes of procedures are explained clearly and fully to the patient, and his voluntary cooperation is enlisted. Procedures are not done *to* a person, but *with* him, with his understanding and agreement. This is the only way to treat people effectively and satisfactorily, and this is the inherent understanding of the behavioral scientist.

REFERENCES

Erickson, M. H.: Further clinical techniques of hypnosis; utilization techniques. *Am J Clin Hypn, 1*:3, 1959.

Hollon, T. H.: Behavior modification in a community rehabilitation unit. *Arch Phys Med Rehabil, 54*:65, 1973.

Hurwitz, R.: Behavior modification with a brain-damaged, antisocial young adult. Unpublished manuscript, 1973.

Kushner, Heraldean and Knox, A. W.: Application of the utilization technique to the behavior of a brain-injured patient. *J Commun Dis, 6*:151, 1973.

Osborne, J. G.: Behavior modification with a deaf student: A case study. *Psychol Asp Disabil, 17*:71, 1970.

Sand, Patricia, L., Trieschmann, Roberta B., Fordyce, W. E. and Fowler, R. S.: Behavior modification in the medical rehabilitation setting: Rationale and some applications. *Rehab Res Pract Rev, 1*:11, 1970.

Taylor, G. P. and Persons, R. W.: Behavior modification techniques in a physical medicine and rehabilitation center. *J Psychol, 74*:117, 1970.

Chapter Nine

THE BEHAVIORAL APPROACH TO PATIENT CARE

SOME OF THE MOST important patient behaviors in a rehabilitation hospital take place on the patients' wards or floors, the patients' actual living areas. This is where patients eat, sleep, dress, wash, toilet, take medication, socialize, and engage in a host of other daily activities. Many of these activities are related directly or indirectly to a patient's health, and problems arising in these areas often have to be dealt with rapidly to prevent serious medical complications or, in some cases, life-threatening consequences. Because of the nature of the difficulties and the environmental location of their occurrence, physicians and nurses frequently need to become involved in the treatment programs designed by the behavioral scientist. The studies presented in this chapter represent a sampling of such endeavors.

IMPROVING HYGIENE AND SELF-CARE BEHAVIORS

Hygiene and self-care are important not only for the outward, physical appearance of a patient and for the promotion of independence in activities of daily living, but neglect of personal cleanliness can lead to serious health problems, such as decubiti. The following case illustrates this fact.

Roberts, Dinsdale, Matthews and Cole (1969) treated a twenty-nine-year-old man who had undergone a hemicorporectomy at the L_5-S_1 level of the spinal cord, posteriorly, and along the iliac crest, anteriorly. The bladder and proximal urethra were attached to a urethrostomy on the abdominal wall below the colostomy opening. Following surgery, the patient developed recurrent wound breakdowns, wound abcesses, decubiti, drug-induced hepatitis and jaundice, and required three successive operations for recurrent squamous cell carcinoma. One- and one-half years post-hemicorporectomy he was discharged from the hospital with a sitting plastic jacket prosthesis which permitted wheelchair mobility in an upright position.

During the next three years, the patient required treatment for twelve separate decubitous ulcers. Eight months later he was readmitted to the rehabilitation hospital for final fitting of a walking prosthesis and gait training, and he learned to ambulate well, independently. While he was hospitalized, areas of skin breakdown developed over the anterior and posterior aspects of the stump, despite constant staff supervision. These recurrent ulcers were considered to be the result of a life-long pattern of uncleanliness. The decision was made to use a behavior modification approach to improve the patient's personal hygiene and thereby reduce the frequency and severity of decubiti.

The general principles of behavior modification were explained to the rehabilitation staff. Then the patient was observed over a period of time in order to determine an appropriate reinforcer. Since he drank a great deal of coffee every day, and since this appeared to be important to him, coffee was selected as the reinforcer.

The following plan then was instituted: The patient's physician wrote an order restricting his coffee intake so that he could have a cup of coffee only if he "bought" it with a dated coupon. The staff constructed a list of twelve desirable hygiene tasks, and the patient could earn one cup of coffee for performing each task daily.

The tasks were as follows:

1. Emptying his urine bag and urine graduate in the morning
2. Emptying his urine bag and urine graduate in the evening
3. Colostomy care and waste disposal
4. Bathing
5. Requesting a change of linen in the morning
6. Requesting a change of linen in the evening
7. Cleaning and lining the prosthesis in the evening
8. Axillary care
9. Cleaning and trimming his nails
10. Brushing his teeth in the morning
11. Brushing his teeth in the evening

12. Shaving

The first seven tasks were related directly to the control of decubitus ulcers and the last five items were added so that the patient's outward appearance would make him more suitable for employment.

The patient was told that his skin care and personal hygiene were a matter of life and death for him. The program was explained to him and he agreed to cooperate. Each time he performed one of the self-care tasks on the list a nurse gave him a coupon dated for the following day. When he presented a coupon he received a cup of coffee, whether at meal times, on his floor, or in a therapy class. Without a coupon he could not obtain coffee. The other patients were informed of the program so that they would not get him coffee without first receiving a coupon from him.

After two months, the program was evaluated as to its effectiveness. It was found that during the two-month period the patient had performed each of the twelve required tasks every day. The data are shown in Figure 9-1.

During the patient's several prolonged hospitalizations, when his hygiene was performed for him by others, there were no skin breakdowns. However, the percentages of decubiti when he was not hospitalized were extraordinarily high, being 100 percent most of the time. The behavior modification program, which required him to be responsible for his own self-care while in the hospital, began in September, 1967. It clearly can be seen that skin breakdowns were zero during this entire period.

When the patient was transferred from the rehabilitation hospital to a nursing home the program was discontinued, but the patient continued to maintain his good self-care behavior, performing all twelve tasks every day. He began working in a sheltered workshop, and was hospitalized for eight weeks for urolithiasis and an intrarenal abscess. Upon his return to the nursing home he continued to care for himself, and a follow-up one year later revealed him to be free of stump irritation and decubiti.

It was obvious to the investigators that the patient's slovenly habits resulted from a lifetime spent in an environment where cleanliness was neither taught nor considered important. In fact,

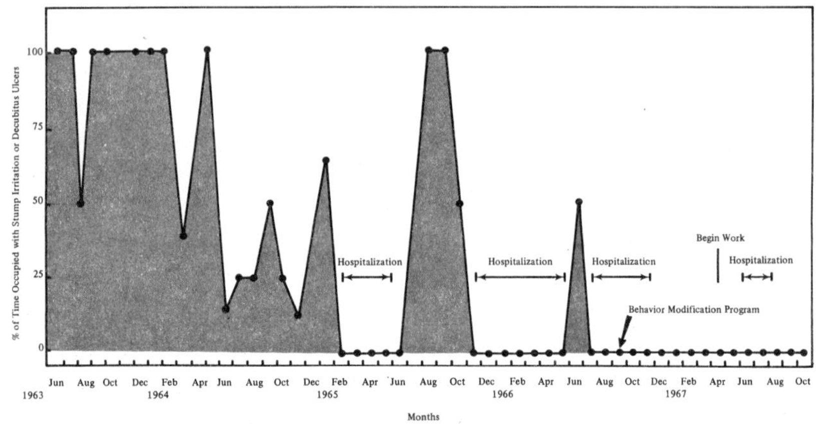

Figure 9-1 Percentage of time confined to bed with stump irritation or decubiti. Incomplete records are shown by dotted lines. From Roberts, A. H., Dinsdale, S. M., Matthews, R. E. and Cole, T. M.: Modifying persistent undesirable behavior in a medical setting. *Arch Phys Med Rehabil, 50*:147, 1969.

Reproduced with the permission of the senior author and the *Archives of Physical Medicine and Rehabilitation.*

poor hygienic practices may have been reinforced by permitting him to do as he wished regardless of his appearance or self-care behaviors. The behavior modification program altered the contingencies so that he could not do as he pleased, i.e. drink coffee, unless he changed his behavior.

The question might legitimately be posed: Why didn't the patient engage in self-care activities for the sake of his own health and as a life saving measure? Wasn't that more important to him than drinking coffee?

The answer to this is, of course, yes, his health and life were more important than a cup of coffee, and his frequent hospitalizations for treatment of decubiti must, at least, have been a source of considerable frustration and annoyance to him and hence a punisher for unclean habits. However, one may also question whether this patient ever directly attributed his skin breakdowns to poor personal hygiene. He had, after all, undergone surgery of the most major proportions, and it is likely that he could have associated the surgery itself, the site of the operation, and the accompanying physical and medical problems with his decubitus ulcers, without realizing the relationship between his own personal care practices and the problem. Since these had become a part of his way of life and his general behavior patterns, he was unlikely to have given the matter much thought, just as he probably gave little thought to drinking coffee.

When something new was introduced into his daily routine, i.e. having to earn his coffee, because it was contingent upon performing certain behaviors, his attention became focussed on those behaviors. In order to obtain something he wanted, which was important to him, he had to perform in certain ways. Thus, a pattern of behaving, which had developed over many years, was interrupted and a new pattern developed. He continued to care for himself even when the contingencies were no longer in effect because new habits had been instated and were being maintained by social reinforcement. As he stated, people were responding more favorably toward him.

* * * * *

Sand, Trieschmann, Fordyce and Fowler (1970) employed a quota-reward system with a twenty-eight-year-old paraplegic man. While in the rehabilitation hospital, he often omitted necessary self-care tasks, or took so long to complete them that he missed his scheduled therapy classes.

The appropriate behaviors which were expected of the patient daily, were as follows:

1. Record pH
2. Record intake and output of fluids
3. Irrigate catheter
4. Take medication
5. Washing
6. Dressing
7. Removing and cleaning urine collection bag
8. Put on braces
9. Be at occupational therapy on time
10. Be at physical therapy on time.

Records were kept, for one week, of the number of items on this list which the patient completed each day. Based upon these records, performance quotas were set, beginning at slightly below the observed baseline frequencies. During each successive week, the expected daily quotas were increased by one. When the patient met the quotas he was reinforced with a weekend pass to visit his home and family.

When the list was introduced, the patient's behavior improved without the addition of the reinforcement contingencies. Satisfactory items per day ranged from 13 to a high of 22, with 22 the total possible. Once quotas were set, the patient began actively participating in all aspects of his rehabilitation program. By the end of the first week of the program he was consistently at, or above 19 of the 22 possible items. This performance was maintained by the patient for four weeks until his transfer to another medical service. He continued to exhibit excellent self-care behavior on the new service despite the fact that the contingency program was discontinued there.

It is interesting to speculate as to the reason for the list alone resulting in improved behavior. One might suppose that the patient actually was unaware of what was expected of him, and the list provided information which he was prepared to utilize since he desired to perform those tasks anyway. A second possible explanation might be that this patient needed a more concrete approach, that verbal instructions were too vague or too abstract, and a formally written list provided him with the necessary structure. Perhaps staff approval followed his performance of the various activities, and this was reinforcing for the patient. There may also have been intrinsic reinforcement in keeping himself clean and healthy, and in acting independently. Finally, one must consider the possibility of a "Hawthorne effect," i.e. merely the fact that he was receiving special attention produced the desired effects.

Since a conclusive explanation is not clear, it also is possible to speculate as to what would have transpired had the quota-reward system not been put into effect. Would the patient's appropriate self-care behaviors have been maintained, or even increased in frequency? Only a replication of the study, with all of the variables controlled, can answer this question.

PREVENTION OF DECUBITI

Among the most serious problems encountered by a patient with a spinal cord injury are decubiti. When a patient remains in one position, such as seated in a wheelchair for an extended period of time, pressure sores can develop over the bony prominences of the body. The lack of nerve supply to the skin makes spinal patients particularly prone to the development of these sores, and they can remain undetected for some time because of the lack of sensation to the involved body area which prevents the patient from knowing that his skin is breaking down. A decubitus ulcer, once developed, can lead to the discontinuation of all rehabilitation therapies until it heals, a process which may require several months. Surgery, such as skin grafting or amputation, and long bed rests are also possible consequences of decubiti, depending upon how advanced the lesions are, the extent of them, the body areas involved, and how long they have progressed undetected. Therefore, prevention of pressure sores is of the utmost importance. Prevention consists, primarily, of intermittent relief of pressure on body areas which are prone to skin breakdown.

An operant conditioning approach to decubitus prevention was utilized by Malament, Dunn and Davis (1974). They used a combination of escape and avoidance conditioning techniques to relieve pressure on the ischium of five patients with spinal cord injuries. The patients could terminate a thirty-second alarm by pushing up from their wheelchair seats after its onset, or they could postpone the onset of the alarm by pushing up before it was activated.

All of the patients in this research were adult males. They were selected for participation because each one had an ischial sore in the process of healing, and none exercised regularly or sufficiently enough to prevent decubiti. Their participation in the experiment was voluntary. Three of the patients had lesions at the lumbar level of the spinal cord, and two had thoracic lesions.

A pressure-sensitive switch was placed under each patient's wheelchair seat cushion. When the patient rose from the seat, the switch opened and started a four-second timer. If the patient remained off the seat for four seconds, a count was made on a cumulative counter which recorded the number of times the patient responded. If the patient sat down before the four-second interval had elapsed, no count was made. If the patient did not rise from the wheelchair seat at least once every ten minutes, a 68-80 db alarm was activated for thirty seconds. The alarm could be postponed for ten minutes if the patient pushed up from the seat before it sounded, or it could be shut off for ten minutes when the patient rose from the seat after it sounded. Each time the alarm was activated it was recorded on an alarm counter.

The training period consisted of three phases.

Phase 1, Baseline Period: During this phase the patients were instructed to go about their daily routine as they usually did. The alarm system was deactivated, but each pushup was recorded on the cumulative counter, and each failure to push up during any ten-minute period was recorded on the alarm counter.

Phase 2, Treatment Period: The patients were informed that an alarm would sound for thirty seconds if a pushup was not executed within every 10-minute period. The alarm system was activated and the patients were instructed to try to prevent the alarm from sounding. Each correct response postponed the onset of the alarm for ten minutes.

Phase 3, Post-Treatment Period: The alarm system was deactivated without the knowledge of the patients. This period was used to assess the effectiveness of the treatment phase. The patients still were under instructions to prevent the alarm from going off. All responses were recorded as before, and after each one-hour session responses were plotted.

The number of sessions in each phase of the study was determined by the daily routines of the patients. Each patient remained in each phase until stability of responding had occurred. The criterion for stability was as follows: The first ten hours of any phase were not considered. For the next ten sessions, the mean of the first five sessions was compared with the mean of the last five sessions. If the difference between means was less than 10 percent of the ten-session mean, the patient was considered to have stabilized in responding and was shifted to the next phase. If the difference between submeans was greater than 10 percent of the grand mean, another experimental session was added and the calculations were performed for that session and the nine sessions immediately preceding it. This procedure was continued until the patient reached the 10 percent criterion.

The criterion for success in the experiment was a patient receiving no more than three alams over a five-session period. (There were a possible thirty alarms which could be received within five sessions.) Advancing to ***Phase 3,*** and finally moving off the program, was contingent upon the criterion for success being met and a stable rate of pushups being achieved.

Two weeks after the completion of the study, two of the patients were followed up in an attempt to evaluate the effectiveness of the training, i.e. if the pushup behavior was being maintained. Their alarms were not activated, but the counters kept records of how often the alarms would have sounded had they been in effect.

Two of the patients were discharged from the hospital after only eight and ten sessions, respectively. They were not on the program long enough for it to have been effective with them, and they lived at too great a distance from the institution to continue the training on an out-patient basis. One patient consistently pushed up from his wheelchair seat every fifteen minutes, and to

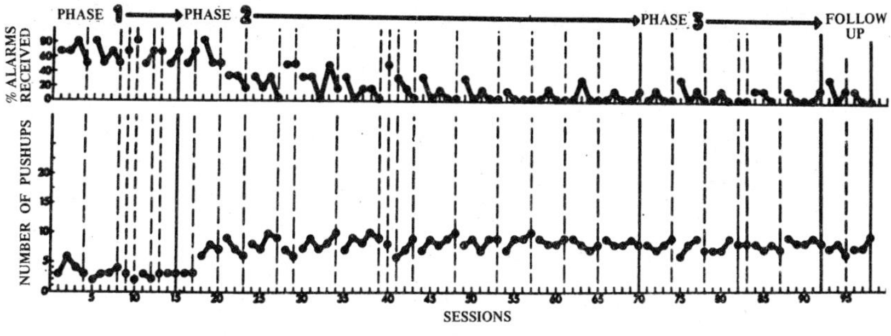

Figure 9-2 Number of pushups and percent alarms received for Case 1 (the fourth patient). From Malament, I. B., Dunn, M. E. and Davis, R.: Pressure sores: An operant conditioning approach to prevention. *Arch Phys Med Rehabil, 56*:161, 1975.

Reproduced with the permission of the senior author and the *Archives of Physical Medicine and Rehabilitation.*

train him to push up every ten minutes would have been uneconomical in terms of time and effort.

Figure 9-2 presents the data for a fourth patient. The upper ordinate shows the percentage of alarms received. The lower plotting indicates the number of pushups performed. The number of sessions is located on the horizontal axis. Data points representing different sessions are connected only when they occurred on the same day.

During the baseline phase, this patient made few pushups and

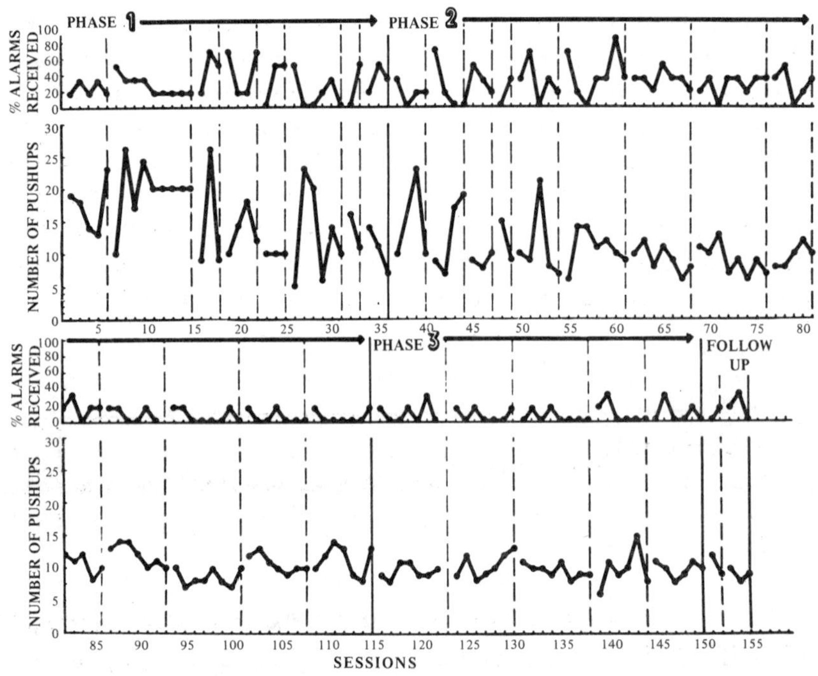

Figure 9-3 Number of pushups and percent alarms received for Case 2 (the fifth patient). From Malament, I. B., Dunn, M. E. and Davis, R.: Pressure sores: An operant conditioning approach to prevention. *Arch Phys Med Rehabil, 56*:161, 1975.

Reproduced with the permission of the senior author and the *Archives of Physical Medicine and Rehabilitation.*

would have received many alarms had the system been activated. ***Phase 2*** data shows a gradual increase in the number of pushups performed, and a corresponding decrease in the number of alarms. Over the last ten sessions of ***Phase 2,*** the patient averaged 8.3 pushups per session with only 6.7 percent alarms. These levels were maintained during ***Phase 3,*** and also upon follow-up two weeks later.

The results of the procedure with the fifth patient are illustrated in Figure 9-3. His baseline performance was highly erratic, varying between five and twenty-seven pushups per session. However, the high rate of pushups did not prevent him from sitting too long. In ***Phase 2*** his behavior became more regular. His pushup rate averaged 10.7 over the final ten sessions of this phase, while the percent alarms he received declined to a mean of 0.3 per session. This responding continued throughout ***Phase 3,*** and was observed to be maintained during the follow-up period.

There is a similarity between the present investigation and the one by Roberts et al., which was discussed at the beginning of this chapter. Both studies were concerned with the formation of new habits. The patient in the earlier mentioned research had spent a lifetime engaging in incorrect hygiene habits, while the subjects in the investigation by Malament et al. had to acquire a habit which they had not engaged in previously to any significant extent. Individuals, as a general rule, do not have the habit of constantly pushing up from their chairs after precise time intervals. While the Roberts et al. procedure had to undo bad habits first, the present researchers had to instill a new one. In both cases, however, the new habits persisted once they had been acquired, as habits are wont to do.

A key feature of the work of Malament and his colleagues is the precision with which they defined their criteria for stability and success. Only with such careful measurement is it possible to proceed accurately from one step of an experiment to the next. Proceeding too slowly is inefficient, and advancing too rapidly can lead to failure. When the investigator has predetermined the criteria for stable responding at each level of the study — baseline, treatment, and termination — he assures himself, as much as possible, of correct procedure. The interested reader can consult

Sidman (1960) for a detailed discussion of these considerations.

ASSURING FLUID INTAKE

The leading causes of premature death among patients with spinal cord injuries are urinary tract and renal infections. In order to minimize the risk of such complications, patients are advised to maintain a high daily fluid intake, usually of approximately 3,000 cc. They are reminded periodically, by their physicians and nurses, of the necessity for this, and records are kept of their daily fluid intake and output through urination.

However, acquiring the habit of drinking this amount of fluid usually is not easy for most patients, and many never achieve the desired goal. The nurse then reports to the physician that a patient's urine output is low and/or highly concentrated. Because of the importance of proper drinking behavior, the staff renews its efforts to explain to the patient the need for a high fluid intake, and to encourage him to drink more than he has been doing. The physician may write an order to "force" fluids. Sometimes this is effective, but sometimes it is not, and even leads to a decrease of fluid intake. This in turn results in greater staff attention to the problem. What can be seen as happening, from a behavioral standpoint, is that greater attention is being given to the patient for not drinking than would be given if he were following instructions.

This typical vicious cycle, as described by Fordyce (1968), has been dealt with through an operant approach to the basic problem by Fowler, Fordyce and Berni (1969).

In their procedure, the nurse gives the patient a notebook or clipboard to keep with him, in which he records his daily fluid intake. This record is made public in the form of a graph. The treatment staff responds positively to increases in drinking by calling attention to them, letting the patient know that they are aware of the difficulty of his task, and praising him. Decreases in drinking are ignored.

An example of the effects of this simple technique can be seen in Figure 9-4. This figure presents the record of a thirty-seven-year-old, paraplegic housewife. She had a long history of poor self-care resulting in frequent medical complications. Although she had

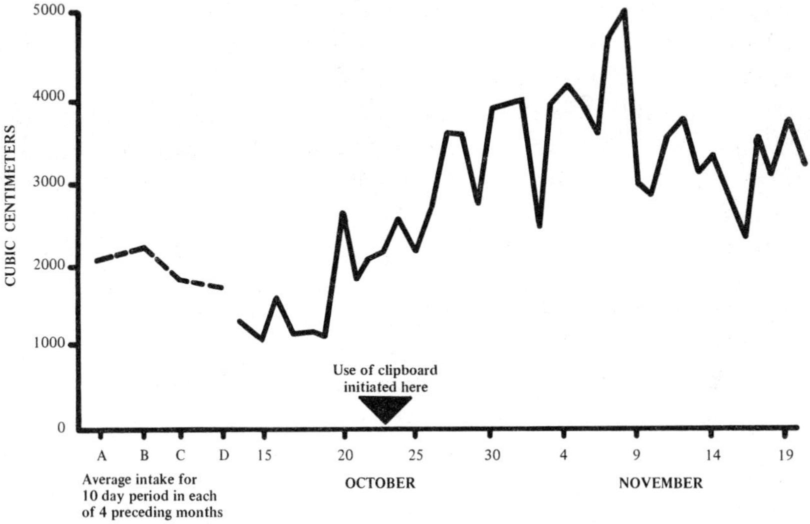

Figure 9-4 Changes in fluid intake as a result of operant treatment. From Fordyce, W. E.: The learning model and psychology's role in medical rehabilitation. Paper presented at the Annual Convention of the American Psychological Association, San Francisco, 1968; and Fowler, R. S., Fordyce, W. E. and Berni, Rosemarian: Operant conditioning in chronic illness. *Am J Nurs, June*:1226, 1969.

Reproduced with the permission of the senior authors, the American Psychological Association and the *American Journal of Nursing*. Copyright June, 1969, The American Journal of Nursing Company.

been advised to drink at least 3,000 cc of fluid per day, she gradually had decreased her fluid intake. The more attention she received for this behavior, the less she drank.

On the figure, points A, B, C, and D represent the means of ten-day samples of her drinking from the four months immediately preceding the start of the operant program. The arrow at October 23 indicates when she was given a clipboard and instructed in its use. It clearly can be seen that her fluid intake was increased significantly. At the time of her discharge, she was maintaining a fluid intake of 3,000 cc daily.

Sand, Trieschmann, Fordyce and Fowler (1970) replicated the procedure with a forty-six-year-old, paraplegic man who had neglected adequate fluid intake for several years. All attempts to inform him of the need for drinking, and to persuade him to drink more, had failed to alter his behavior.

At the beginning of the third week of his hospitalization, bar graphs which showed his daily fluid intake were posted in his room, and he was instructed by the nurses on how to keep his own records. This graphic display provided the patient with immediate feedback of the adequacy and consistency of his fluid intake. In addition, physicians, nurses and psychologists favorably commented and praised him when the graphs showed increased drinking.

The results of the procedures are illustrated in Figure 9-5. It is obvious that the techniques employed markedly increased the patient's fluid intake from the first week in which they were employed.

While these studies make it appear obvious that only informing patients of the necessity for increasing their fluid intake does not lead to the desired behavior, while a behavior modification approach does have such an effect, such a conclusion requires experimental testing to be definitive.

* * * * *

Sand, Fordyce and Fowler (1973) followed up their clinical experiences with an investigation which compared groups of spinal cord-injured patients with regard to increasing their fluid intake.

Ninety-three patients were divided into two groups. Sixty-nine patients received an informational approach, i.e. verbal explanations from physicians and nurses of the importance of drinking large amounts of fluids, and twenty-four patients were treated with behavioral methods as described in the two studies previously discussed.

Data collected over the ten-week period of the study showed that those patients who had a low initial daily fluid output and received information only, continued to have a low fluid output.

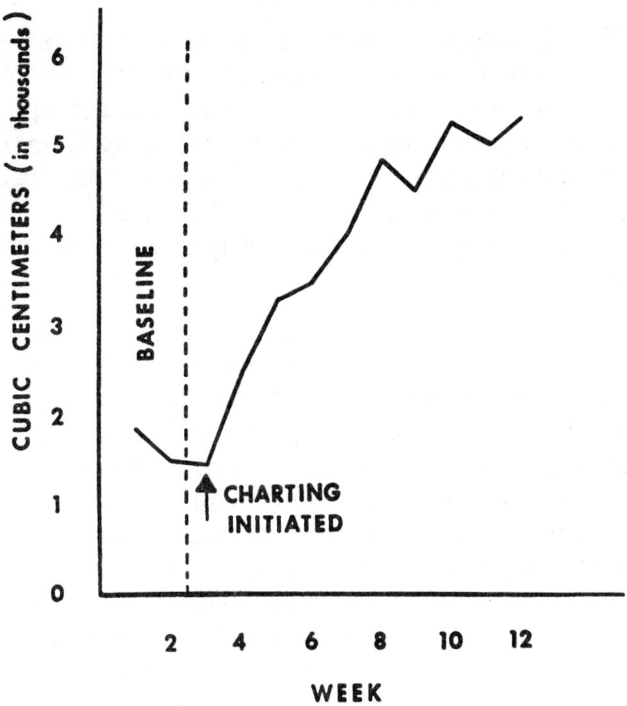

Figure 9-5 Increase in fluid intake for a forty-six-year-old paraplegic as a consequence of behavioral procedures. From Sand, Patricia L., Trieschmann, Roberta B., Fordyce, W. E. and Fowler, R. S.: Behavior modification in the medical rehabilitation setting: Rationale and some applications. *Rehab Res Pract Rev, 1*:11, 1970.

Reproduced with the permission of the senior author and the *Rehabilitation Research and Practice Review*, Arkansas Rehabilitation Research and Training Center.

Those patients whose problem was treated with behavior modification methods significantly increased their daily fluid output.

The conclusion, therefore, which can be drawn from these results is that behavior modification techniques are highly superior to informational methods for increasing drinking behavior in patients with spinal cord injuries.

BLADDER TRAINING

Significant damage to the spinal cord at or above the sacral area invariably leads to bladder incontinence. In the case of a lower motor neuron lesion, the bladder retains urine, expands, and becomes flaccid, resulting in overflow dribbling. The risk of infection is high, and therefore many procedures have been developed in an attempt to treat this condition. These procedures, however, frequently do not meet with complete success. Fazio (1973) employed a functional analysis approach in dealing with this type of problem.

A twenty-two-year-old man, paraplegic as the result of a fall, had a flaccid, neurogenic bladder. During the seven months of his hospitalization, his indwelling catheter had been removed periodically to assess his ability to void independently, but he was unable to do so completely. During the next five months, his voiding ability improved slightly, but due to increased intravesical pressure and high residual urine when he was not catheterized, his physician proposed a transurethral section of either the bladder neck, the prostate, or both. At this point, the patient sought the aid of a psychologist who felt that successful voiding might be facilitated by the use of exteroceptive eliciting or discriminative stimuli. Having good voluntary control over bladder contractions, the aim of a program would be the relaxation of the urinary sphincters and contraction of the bladder on cue.

After a history of the problem had been obtained, detailed descriptions of the problem behaviors and the goals of the treatment program were prepared.

The patient then was instructed to keep a written record of his voiding behavior, and of all stimuli which he considered to be related to his urination. These included the locations in which he urinated, fluid intake, straining, etc. The record was kept for twenty-five days.

The patient had learned from experience that the sensation of a slight "tug" on the bladder was associated with complete voiding. This sensation, therefore, was used to judge the successfulness of his attempts to void.

After the third day, the patient began a fixed pattern of behavior associated with voiding attempts. He would drink seven ounces of cold water, step to the commode, lower his trousers and underwear, and simultaneously stimulate his anus digitally and strain, i.e. contract his diaphragm. Any resulting stream of urine was directed into the commode so that it produced as much noise as possible.

During the first month of this procedure the patient voided completely between 70 and 80 percent of the time. One month later, he was voiding 100 percent of the time, as determined from the sensation of the "tug" on his bladder when he urinated. In addition, he had discontinued drinking the cold water and stimulating his anus, and the straining was more relaxed. It appeared as if the patient spontaneously had recovered the ability to void completely upon desire, since no specific behavior modification techniques had been utilized. The sound of the urine in the water of the commode, however, seemed to be of significance.

Fazio then attempted to evaluate the extent to which exteroceptive stimuli might be functioning in maintaining a steady stream of urine once the stream had been initiated by the patient's straining. A second log of observations was kept for this purpose over a two month period.

Four conditions were tested: sight and sound of the urinary stream; sight of the urinary stream alone; sound of the urinary stream alone; and neither sight nor sound of the urinary stream. The response topography was modified in that no water was drunk just before attempts at voiding, no anal stimulation was employed, and the patient sat on the commode, rather than urinating while standing at it. Straining still was used to initiate the urinary stream, but with reduced effect.

The visual and auditory cues were altered by having the patient either look, or not look at the urinary stream, and by either directing the stream into the water, or against the wall of the bowl.

The four conditions were ordered in random sequence over eighty-six trials. The number of trials per day varied between zero and six, depending upon the completeness of the patient's voidings. The patient kept a record of the results of his voiding attempts, his food and water intake, and the stimulus condition for each attempt.

Auditory	Visual	
	V	V̄
A	23/23 100%	18/19 95%
Ā	15/22 68%	0/22 0%

Note: A = auditory condition (i.e., directing the stream into the water), A = nonauditory (i.e., directing the stream against the wall of the commode to minimize sounds); V = visual; V = nonvisual (i.e., not watching the steadiness of the stream nor its termination).

Table 9-I Percentage of complete voidings by condition. From Fazio, A. F.: The use of functional analysis techniques in bladder training associated with a flaccid neurogenic bladder condition: A case study. *Rehab Psychol, 20*:175, 1973.

Reproduced with the permission of the author and *Rehabilitation Psychology*.

The results, as indicated in Table 9-I, were that auditory stimuli (A) were more closely associated with complete voiding than were visual stimuli (V). (The data revealed that neither success nor failure of an attempt to void were dependent upon an empty or a full bladder.) The combination of auditory and visual cues resulted in 100 percent voiding, while auditory cues alone produced 95 percent voiding. Visual cues alone resulted in 68 percent voiding. When neither auditory nor visual cues were present the percentage of complete voidings was zero.

This study made no use of specific conditioning procedures, although it can be said to have made effective use of naturally occurring conditioning stimuli. Its significance lies in the functional analysis made of the patient's voiding behavior, which determined the environmental and cue conditions under which complete voiding occurred. It remains speculative whether other patients with similar problems can be helped in this way, but it appears to be a possibility. Once the stimuli that are associated with voiding behavior are determined, these stimuli might be utilized as cues to elicit the desired responding.

* * * * *

Ince, Brucker and Alba (1975) employed a classical conditioning paradigm in an experiment designed to bring the reflex arc in the sacral portion of the spinal cord, which controls micturition, under the control of an external stimulus.

Two males, aged thirty-seven and thirty-two years, were seen as subjects. The first subject, L. F., had suffered a transsection of the spinal cord at the T_7-T_8 level as the result of a gunshot wound three years prior to being included in the study. The second subject, A. D., sustained a spinal cord injury at the L_1-L_2 level due to a fall nine months before being seen by the researchers. Both subjects had complete spinal cord transsections and both had spastic neurogenic bladders. The first subject was using a Foley catheter at the beginning of the investigation, and later switched to a condom drainage system. The other subject used condom drainage from the start.

Electrical stimulation of the lower abdomen served as the unconditioned stimulus (UCS) to elicit the unconditioned response (UCR) of urination. The stimulation produced contraction of the abdominal muscles, which increased bladder pressure and initiated voiding. The electrical stimulation was delivered by a sixty-cycle constant voltage shocker, integrated into a programmable unit capable of delivering a preselected current at a specified time for a predetermined duration. A response clock, integrated with the circuitry, was initiated automatically with the presentation of the electrical stimulation, and was stopped by the experimenter when the urinary stream began, thus recording the latency of the response. The abdominal stimulation was delivered through disposable, adhesive, surface electrodes. Electrode jelly was employed to enhance conduction.

The conditioned stimulus (CS) was a mild electrical stimulus applied to the inner surface of the thigh. The stimulus was delivered from a small, hand-held, battery-operated device, with two flat plates on one side which served as electrodes when applied to the skin. A small button, located on the top of the unit, activated the stimulus. The initiation and duration of the CS was governed by signals from the programming unit, which integrated this stimulus with the UCS and the response clock. The subjects' urinary output during the experimental sessions was measured after each trial by a Uri-Meter® (Davol) attached to the catheter drainage tube.

Both subjects were placed on a schedule of drinking 240 cc of water every hour from time of arising to time of retiring. Over a two week period, a baseline measure was obtained of both the frequency of their voiding, and the amount voided each time. Each subject had a calibrated urine collection bag which they checked hourly, and after each observation, each recorded the amount of urine in the bag on special data sheets.

Subjects were seen individually for thirty-minute sessions, five days per week. Each session consisted of between ten and fifteen trials, depending upon the amount of urine excreted within the session. The first session was used to determine the amount of current necessary to produce visible abdominal contractions; once a level was established for each subject, it was maintained throughout the study.

In order to establish the neutrality of the CS, two sessions of fifteen trials each were conducted with both subjects, wherein the CS alone was presented. A trial consisted of the subject pushing up from his wheelchair seat and the experimenter applying the CS to the inner thigh for three seconds. Following these sessions, a series of sessions involving presentation of the UCS alone were conducted in order to establish a reliable voiding response prior to pairing the CS with the UCS. The subject raised himself from the sitting position, and the UCS was delivered to the lower abdomen at the predetermined current level. The onset and the termination of the UCS was regulated automatically by the programming unit. The duration of the UCS was two- and one-half seconds. At the first sign of urination, the clock was stopped and the latency of response was recorded. When the urinary stream ceased, the amount voided was recorded. Each trial was followed by a forty-five second rest interval. Subject L. F. received ninety trials of the UCS, and A. D. received thirty UCS trials.

The conditioning phase of the experiment followed. The CS was applied to the subject's inner thigh one-half second before the onset of the UCS, and both stimuli ran concurrently and terminated simultaneously. The CS had a total duration of three seconds, the last two- and one-half seconds being paired with the UCS. The timing, recording, and resting procedures were the same as during the previous phase of the study. The subjects continued to push up from their wheelchair just prior to stimulation.

Subject L. F. received seven conditioning sessions and subject A. D. received twelve sessions. Trials during which the CS alone was presented were interspersed with the conditioning trials. As the CS began to elicit voiding in the absence of the UCS, the number of CS trials per session were gradually increased, while the number of pairing trials was decreased.

Following the conditioning phase, additional sessions, consisting of CS trials only, were conducted to determine the success of the pairing procedure. Subject L. F. received twelve sessions, while subject A. D. participated in seventeen such sessions.

Upon completion of this phase, L. F., who had been using a Foley catheter, changed to a condom drainage system, and the entire procedure was repeated with him.

Once the CS had been established as an effective stimulus for eliciting urination with both subjects, a shaping procedure was implemented. At first, the subjects pushed up from their wheelchair seats with their arms fully extended. Then, gradually, they pushed up less and less during each session, until finally, they were seated during stimulation. Several trials also were conducted with the subjects seated on a bedpan or commode while receiving the CS, and all CS applications were performed by the subjects themselves when they were in the sitting position.

An analysis of baseline data revealed that A. D. urinated a mean of 54.5 cc per hour, and L. F. had a mean output of 118.4 cc of urine per hour. The results of the two initial CS sessions showed that no voiding responses were elicited from either subject on any trial, indicating that the CS was a neutral stimulus at the beginning of the experiment.

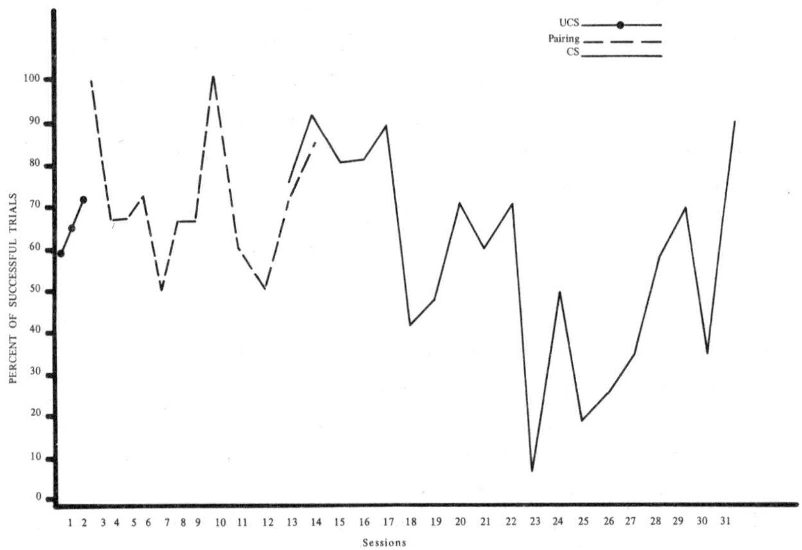

Figure 9-6 Percent of trials eliciting voiding response in the UCS, pairing and CS conditions for Subject A.D. From Ince, L. P., Brucker, B. S. and Alba, A.: Conditioning techniques as a method for bladder control in patients with spinal cord injuries. Paper presented at the Annual Session of the American Congress of Rehabilitation Medicine, Atlanta, 1975.

Reproduced with the permission of the American Congress of Rehabilitation Medicine.

Figure 9-6 shows the percentage of successful trials within each session for the UCS, CS-UCS pairing, and terminal CS conditions for A. D. It can be seen that the UCS successfully elicited voiding approximately 68 percent of the time. The mean latency for these responses was 4.5 seconds. The success rate for the pairing phase was about the same, but the latency was slightly longer for responses during this condition, being 4.7 seconds, on the average. When the CS alone was delivered after the conditioning sessions, the percentage of successful responses remained at approximately the same level. This indicates that the previously neutral CS was eliciting voiding at about the same rate as the UCS. The mean latency for the CS trials was 10.5 seconds. The slightly lower percentages of successful voiding on the later trials occurred when the subject was sitting on a bedpan or a commode.

There was considerable variability in the amount of urine voided by this subject during each session. During the UCS condition it varied between 150 cc and 450 cc. During the pairing sessions, he voided between 25 cc and 375 cc. The subject's output for the sessions in which he received the CS alone was between 10 cc and 475 cc. It should be pointed out, however, that despite the

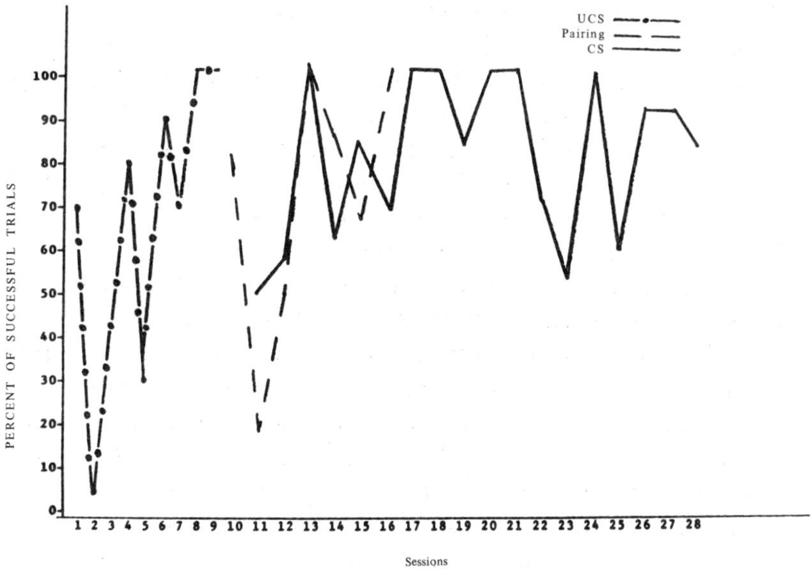

Figure 9-7 Percent of trials eliciting voiding response in the UCS, pairing and CS conditions for Subject L. F. on catheter. From Ince, L. P., Brucker, B. S. and Alba, A.: Conditioning techniques as a method for bladder control in patients with spinal cord injuries. Paper presented at the Annual Session of the American Congress of Rehabilitation Medicine, Atlanta, 1975.

Reproduced with the permission of the American Congress of Rehabilitation Medicine.

differences in output between sessions, he almost always voided more during the experimental sessions than his baseline hourly output of 54.5 cc.

The percentage of successful trials, within each session, for the experimental conditions for L. F. while on Foley catheter drainage is presented in Figure 9-7. Inspection of the graph reveals that the UCS was successful in eliciting voiding. His mean latency of responding under this condition was 10.6 seconds. The pairing trials showed approximately the same rate of success in producing micturition. The average latency for the pairing condition was 6.7 seconds. The CS trials resulted in a highly successful rate of responding, demonstrating again the effectiveness of the previously neutral stimulus. This demonstrated that urination could be conditioned with an indwelling catheter present.

The amount of urine voided by this subject during each session was substantially lower than for the other subject for all experimental conditions because his catheter was a continual drainage device which did not permit urine to collect in the bladder in large amounts. This subject voided a high of 325 cc during the UCS condition, and varied in his output during the pairing and CS conditions between zero and 45 cc per session.

Figure 9-8 shows the percentage of successful trials for the various experimental conditions for subject L. F. when he was on condom drainage. Initially, the UCS did not produce urination, but by the fifth session voiding responses were obtained reliably. The mean latency of these responses was 10.4 seconds. The pairing trials produced a slightly higher rate of success, and had a lower average latency of 6.2 seconds. The CS reliably elicited micturition in the absence of the UCS with a good rate of success. The mean latency of responding was 8.24 seconds.

Considerable variability occurred in the amount of urine voided from session to session. During the UCS condition, output ranged from 50 cc to 650 cc. The subject voided between zero and 650 cc during the conditioning phase, and between zero and 600 cc when the CS was used in the absence of the UCS. As was true with subject A. D., most experimental sessions resulted in higher urine output than the subject's baseline rate.

This study demonstrates that it is possible to condition a

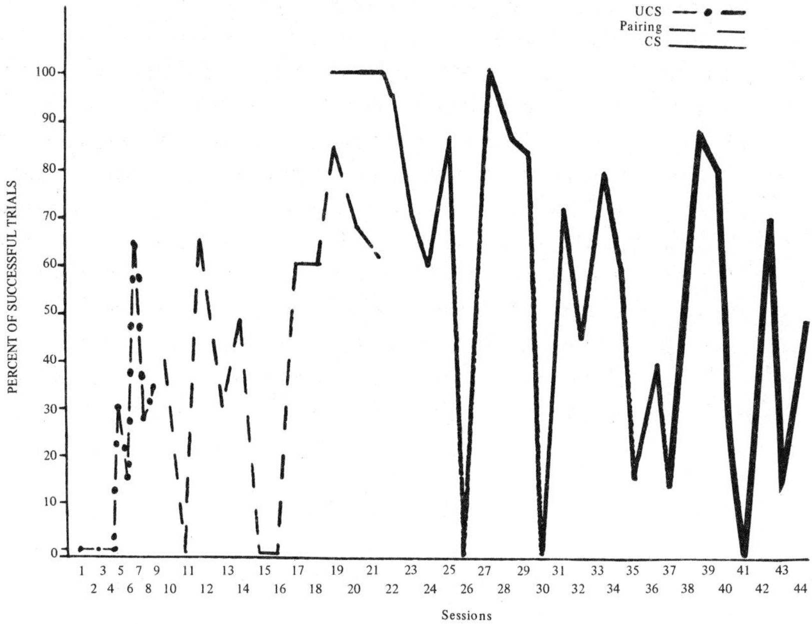

Figure 9-8 Percent of trials eliciting voiding response in the UCS, pairing and CS conditions for Subject L. F. on condom drainage. From Ince, L. P., Brucker, B. S. and Alba, A.: Conditioning techniques as a method for bladder control in patients with spinal cord injuries. Paper presented at the Annual Session of the American Congress of Rehabilitation Medicine, Atlanta, 1975.

Reproduced with the permission of the American Congress of Rehabilitation Medicine.

response which occurs below the level of a spinal cord lesion. Conditioning occurred, with both subjects, in the absence of cognition and brain control. Both the UCS and the CS were delivered below the level of the patients' lesions, indicating responding through spinal cord mechanisms alone. Whether bladder musculature contraction, or the reflex controlling sphincter function was the critical variable which was conditioned cannot conclusively be stated, but it is most probable that the latter was the case. Further investigation is required to determine precisely how the voiding response was experimentally controlled. The fact that a response could be conditioned in the spinal cord in the absence of brain regulation has important implications for neurophysiological theory as well as for practical applications.

An advanced step in a project of this nature would be to have the patients carry the CS device with them and stimulate themselves on a regularly scheduled basis. If the CS continues to elicit urination, with low residual urine and without leakage between stimulations, it appears feasible that such patients could be made independent in bladder functioning, i.e. be able to void upon desire. This would mean the possible total elimination of the need for catheterization or any urinary drainage and collection system, thereby not only avoiding inconvenience and embarrassment but preventing infection and subsequent problems of the urinary system. At present, this possibility remains speculative, but the investigators are continuing their research with that goal in mind.

REFERENCES

Fazio, A. F.: The use of functional analysis techniques in bladder training associated with a flaccid neurogenic bladder condition: A case study. *Rehab Psychol, 20,* 175, 1973.

Fordyce, W. E.: The learning model and psychology's role in medical rehabilitation. Paper presented at the Annual Convention of the American Psychological Association, San Francisco, 1968.

Fowler, R. S., Fordyce, W. E. and Berni, Rosemarian: Operant conditioning in chronic illness. *Am J Nurs, 69,* 1226, 1969.

Ince, L. P., Brucker, B. S. and Alba, Augusta: Conditioning techniques as a method for bladder control in patients with spinal cord injuries. Paper presented at the Annual Session of the American Congress of Rehabilitation Medicine, Atlanta, 1975.

Malament, I. B., Dunn, M. E. and Davis, R.: Pressure sores: An operant conditioning approach to prevention. *Arch Phys Med Rehab, 56*:161, 1975.

Roberts, A. H., Dinsdale, S. M., Matthews, R. E. and Cole, T. M.: Modifying persistent undesirable behavior in a medical setting. *Arch Phys Med Rehab, 50*:147, 1969.

Sand, Patricia L., Fordyce, W. E. and Fowler, R. S.: Fluid intake behavior in patients with spinal cord injury: Prediction and modification. *Arch Phys Med Rehab, 54*:254, 1973.

Sand, Patricia L., Trieschmann, Roberta B., Fordyce, W. E. and Fowler, R. S.: Behavior modification in the medical rehabilitation setting: Rationale and some applications. *Rehab Res Pract Rev, 1*:11, 1970.

Sidman, M.: *Tactics of Scientific Research.* New York, Basic Books, 1960.

Chapter Ten

OPERANT TECHNIQUES IN THE MANAGEMENT OF CHRONIC PAIN

ACCORDING TO STERNBACH (1968), pain is an abstract concept which refers to: 1) a personal, private sensation of hurt, 2) a harmful stimulus which signals current or impending tissue damage, and 3) a pattern or responses which operate to protect the organism from harm.

These responses can be described in several languages: the neurological, which refers to nervous system changes occurring in response to painful stimulation; the physiological, or the peripheral indicants of autonomic nervous system responses; the behavioral, or the bodily responses consequential to pain; and the affective, or subjective, emotional and phenomenal experience of pain.

Pain is conceived of as being both physical and psychological, and these variables interact with each other, making a clearcut distinction difficult.

Pain also is a set of responses. That is, a person must respond in some way to a painful stimulus, external or internal, for an observer to determine that he is experiencing pain.

In rehabilitation, pain can present significant problems. If severe enough, it prevents an affected patient from participating in therapeutic, social and recreational activities. It reduces motivation. It depresses affect. It results in irritability and irascibility. It presents ward management difficulties. It interferes with self-care and ADL behaviors. It requires additional medical and nursing staff time and effort. It interferes with routine functioning. It causes sorrow. Hence, it must be dealt with.

The majority of pain problems encountered in a rehabilitation setting are of a chronic rather than of an acute nature. Included among these problems are the shoulder-hand syndromes of hemiplegic patients; the phantom limb pains of amputees; contractures, spasms, thalamic syndromes; the joint pains of patients with rheumatoid arthritis; chronic low back pains; hyperaesthesias; and many others, some of which are disability-specific, such as the gas pains experienced by quadriplegic patients.

There are numerous medical procedures which are employed in the treatment of pain, primarily chemotherapy and surgery. These often are effective, but also frequently are of limited permanent value. This chapter examines the concept of chronic pain from a psychological viewpoint and presents the behavioral approach to treatment.

Fordyce (1974a) contrasts the medical, or disease model, of pain with the psychological or behavioral model. (For a thorough description and discussion of these models as applied to psychological problems in general, the reader should consult Ullmann and Krasner, 1965.)

The medical model considers pain as an event which is under the control of some underlying pathology. Diagnoses are aimed at uncovering this pathology, and treatment is designed to eliminate the cause and not the symptom of the pain. If diagnostic procedures fail to identify a sufficient organic cause, or if organically-based treatment methods do not resolve the pain problem, the pain often becomes viewed as psychogenic, hypochondriacal, or malingering. In such a case, the patient may be referred for psychotherapy. Or, he may be told that there is nothing wrong with him and he will have to learn to live with the pain. Thus the inferred underlying pathology has been shifted from some body tissue to the brain, and the antecedent stimulus is presumed to reside in the patient's "psyche." The pain still is viewed in medical model terms.

The behavioral model presents an alternative. Its basic proposition is that behavior, including pain behavior, is learned. That which the medical model considers to be symptoms, the behavioral model views as behavior which is under the control of environmental consequences. In other words, pain is an operant. The initial determination, therefore, to be made when a patient presents a pain problem or engages in pain behavior is of the environmental phenomena which are controlling the pain behaviors. An analysis is made of the relationships between the occurrence of pain behavior and the consequences of that behavior in the patient's environment.

Since the stimuli which produce pain are unobservable, inferences about pain are made from the auditory and visual cues presented by the patient, such as moans, complaints, grimaces, guarded movements and functional impairments. All of these behaviors are operants and are subject to influence by their consequences. It logically is assumed that these pain behaviors have come to be controlled by learning factors. If this is so, there is no need to consider the existence of underlying pathology to account for the pain behaviors.

When a patient exhibits pain, it is quite likely that his pain behaviors will be followed by reinforcing consequences. Among these reinforcers are medications, which are given contingent upon expressions of pain and the need for relief; rest from activity, permitted when the patient complains of pain; attention from physicians and nurses; and solicitous remarks and attention from others. Unless there is pain behavior, these reinforcers will not be given to the patient.

Pain is a punishing experience, and it is known that behavior which successfully avoids punishment tends to increase in frequency. It would be expected, therefore, that chronic pain could control the behavior of a patient far beyond that which would be anticipated as a direct result of the occurrence of similar pain stimuli on a temporary or transient basis. The patient seeks out situations where the probability of experiencing pain is as low as possible. Chronic pain can cause some individuals to learn to overreact and restrict their activities in a way that constitutes a serious disability or functional impairment beyond that actually caused by the pain. If the behaviors in which the patient engages were previously successful in avoiding or reducing pain, they have a high probability of continuing even when pain no longer is present.

In sum, pain behaviors may be reinforced directly by medication, rest and attention, all environmental consequences which are contingent upon the pain. Additionally, many alleged pain behaviors are responses which have been developed over time to avoid pain and continue to occur in the absence of pain.

Once an evaluation of the patient's situation has determined that the pain behaviors are under the control of environmental consequences, the treatment focuses on behavior change. This change consists of the reduction of pain behaviors and the increase of well behaviors.

From a behavioral approach to pain, Fordyce (1974b) has developed a treatment plan based upon operant learning principles. The plan has three main strategies. The *first* is that pain behaviors may be reduced by withdrawing positive reinforcement from them. The *second* is that well behaviors can be increased by making positive reinforcement contingent upon them. The *third* is that, if gains made in treatment are to be maintained, the natural environment of the patient must be rearranged in order to modify the consequences to sick and well behaviors existing therein.

There are four major components to this general program: patient selection, medication, exercise-activity level and attention.

Patient Selection. The criteria for a patient who has pain to be treated with behavioral techniques are the following: a) No, minimal, or speculative presence of organic pathology; b) A functional analysis indicates that pain behaviors are being reinforced systematically and well behaviors are not receiving reinforcement; c) The reinforcers of medication, rest, and attention appear to effectively be influencing the patient's behavior; d) It appears feasible to bring about sufficient changes in the patient's natural environment that treatment gains will be maintained by the absence of reinforcement for pain behaviors and the delivery of reinforcement for well behaviors; and e) The patient and his/her family agree to participate in the treatment program.

Medication. Instead of giving the patient medication when he asks for it, the medication is delivered on a time-contingent basis independent of how the patient feels. By doing this, medication no longer can be a reinforcer contingent upon pain behavior.

Initially, a baseline of medication requirements is obtained. The patient is observed for several days to determine how much medication he takes, how frequently he takes it, and the time intervals between doses. Once these are known, the patient's medications are put on a time schedule such that the interval between doses is slightly shorter than baseline observations showed his needs to be. For example, if a patient had been requesting medication on a five-hour schedule, the doses are placed on a four-hour schedule. Medications are delivered around the clock, regardless of whether or not the patient expresses a need for them. Then, the level of active ingredients in the medication vehicle gradually is reduced. This is done over a period of seven or eight weeks to avoid acute withdrawal symptoms.

Exercise-Activity Level. Many patients who have chronic pain restrict their physical activities in order to avoid pain, and those around the patient tend to promote this avoidance behavior. The patient's physician may prescribe rest, contingent upon the pain. The patient's physical therapist may encourage him to cease activity and rest when he experiences pain, making rest and therapist attention contingent upon complaints of hurting.

In modifying this situation, the initial step is the observation of the patient in his activities. He is asked to engage in those exercises which, if carried out, would lead eventually to pain. When the patient's tolerance is known, contingencies are rearranged so that rest (and attention from the therapist) does not occur following pain, but instead occurs following activity or exercise.

The patient is assigned a quota for each exercise, beginning at quotas below his demonstrated tolerance limit. This insures that rest will occur prior to pain and immediately after exercise. The quotas gradually are increased according to a predetermined schedule and are not dependent upon the patient's feelings. When a patient fails to meet a particular quota it is reduced and then gradually is increased again.

Attention. Typically, a patient's complaints of pain are responded to by others with sympathy and attempts to help. Even when mild complaints are ignored initially, or responded to negatively, if the patient signals intense pain others try to become helpful and solicitous. Thus, environmental consequences, including attention from physicians and nurses, tend to be positively reinforcing. When the patient does not express pain, on the other hand, he does not receive this attention from people.

The objective of a behavioral approach is to let attention and responsiveness be contingent upon well behaviors and not upon pain responses. The patient's signals of pain are to be ignored or greeted by others as impassively as possible. In addition to the hospital staff responding to the patient in this way, his family members are instructed regarding how to alter the manner in which they respond to the patient.

Basically, this represents the behavioral approach to the problem of chronic pain. It is of interest now to examine some research and case studies where this methodology has been applied.

* * * * *

Fordyce, Fowler and DeLateur (1968) treated the chronic low back pain of a thirty-seven-year-old, married woman. She had experienced constant, aching pain in her lower back for eighteen years, which was made more severe by activity. She had become increasingly unable to carry out her normal homemaking activities, and could work only for approximately twenty minutes without requiring rest. Episodes of pain resulted in the cessation of all activity, resting on a bed or a couch, taking pain medication, and weeping until the pain subsided. The patient had undergone four separate surgical procedures, none of which had been successful in eliminating the pain. A careful neurological examination had revealed no neurologic deficit nor signs of nerve root irritation.

When she was admitted to the rehabilitation hospital, the patient was taking four or five habit-forming analgesic tablets per day, ingesting one tablet each time she experienced pain. Her medication regimen was changed to a time-based schedule of delivery. Medication was given regularly, on a twenty-four-hour basis, regardless of whether or not she complained of pain. A taste and color masking vehicle was added to the medication, and once the regimen had been established, the narcotic content of the medication was decreased gradually without the patient's knowledge. By the fortieth day of her hospitalization, the narcotic content had been eliminated completely from all of her medication. Following this, the doses were decreased to a four-hour schedule, eliminating the usual midnight dose.

All treatment staff, including physicians, nurses, aides and therapists, were instructed to be as neutral and unresponsive as possible when the patient complained of pain and discomfort. When she was observed participating in an activity, the staff was to be friendly and socially responsive, and to lavishly praise daily increases in her level of activity.

In occupational therapy, the patient was given the task of weaving on a standard floor loom. This work required considerable movement of her extremities, and had to be performed in a standing position, one which she had described previously as being extremely painful for her. She was instructed to work as long as she could, and a baseline measure was obtained of approximately twenty-five threads per twenty-minute activity tolerance. Then she was told that she had to add ten threads each day to her previous day's total before she would be permitted to leave occupational therapy and return to her ward for a rest.

By the thirteenth day, the patient had completed weaving a large tablecloth, and was working continuously for more than sixty minutes at a time. By the thirtieth day, she had completed several projects in occupational therapy and was working steadily for two hours, the full class period.

The patient also was given a program of ambulation in physical therapy. She was assigned a daily schedule of walking 200-foot laps around her ward in the morning, and again in the afternoon. Her baseline performance was approximately ten laps before she complained of pain which was intolerable, or fatigue requiring rest.

She was begun at sets of ten laps in the morning and ten more in the afternoon. She was instructed to report to the ward nurses at the outset, and again upon completion of her ambulation. The nurses reinforced the desired behavior. Reinforcement consisted of social attention and praise, rest, and her own record, which she kept in a small notebook. Every ten days, the patient was instructed to increase the number of laps in each set by five.

After seven weeks, the patient was ambulating twenty-five laps, for a total of 5,000 feet, both morning and afternoon, taking the same amount of time that it initially had taken her to walk only ten laps. Figure 10-1 presents this data.

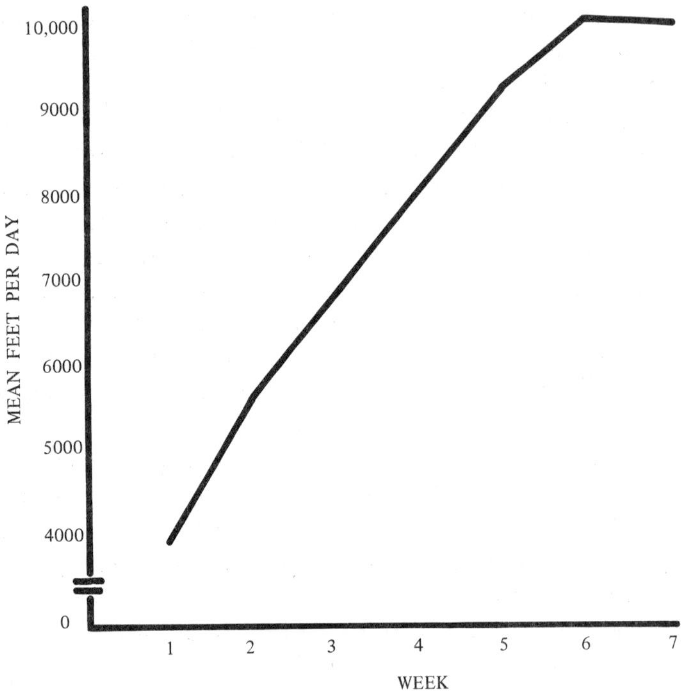

Figure 10-1 Mean daily walking distance by week. From Fordyce, W. E., Fowler, R. S., Lehmann, J. F. and DeLateur, Barbara: Some implications of learning in problems of chronic pain. *J Chronic Dis, 21*:179, 1968.
Reproduced with the permission of the senior author and the *Journal of Chronic Disease*. Copyright 1968, Pergamon Press.

The patient's husband had reported that prior to the start of the behavior modification program she had spent approximately two hours per day in nonreclining activities. He was asked to keep a record of the amount of time she now spent in nonreclining activities, and he was instructed also in ways of being nonresponsive to pain behaviors and reinforcing well behaviors. The records were kept by the patient's husband during her weekends at home, and following her discharge to an out-patient program.

Figure 10-2 illustrates the total number of hours per week that

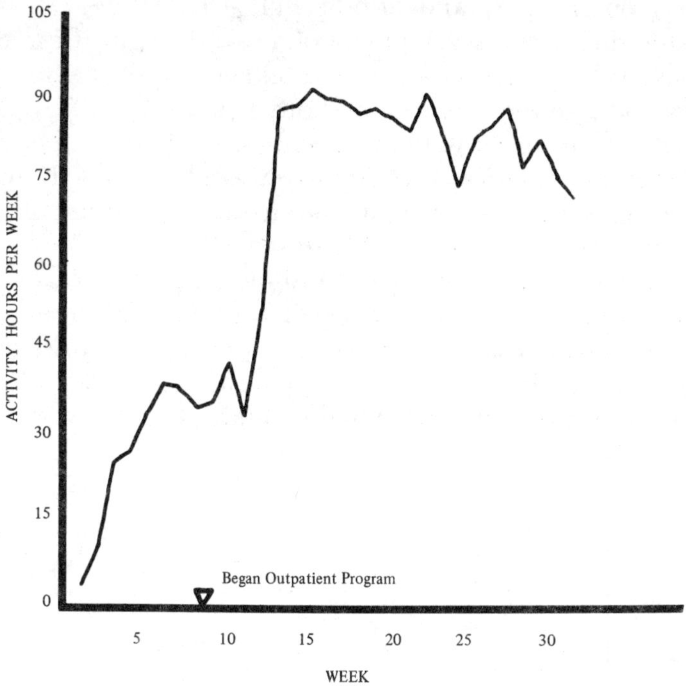

Figure 10-2 Hours of nonreclining activity per week. From Fordyce, W. E., Fowler, R. S. and DeLateur, Barbara: An application of behavior modification technique to a problem of chronic pain. *Behav Res Ther, 6*:105, 1968.

Reproduced with the permission of the senior author and *Behaviour Research and Therapy*. Copyright 1968, Pergamon Press.

the patient spent in nonreclining activities. It is clear that from the beginning of the operant program this increased markedly. Upon her discharge there was a brief return to complaining about pain and a decrease in activity, but she soon returned to her new, high level. The family acquired a second car and the patient became independently mobile in the community.

* * * * *

A second example of behavioral techniques applied to a pain problem is provided by the study of Fordyce, Fowler, Lehmann and DeLateur (1968).

The patient was a forty-six-year-old, married man with a six-year history of intractible back pain. He had had five operations, including a laminectomy, diskectomy, two fusions of the spinal column, one at L_5-S_1, and the other at L_4 -L_5, plus a refusion of the latter due to the development of a pseudoarthrosis, multiple lumbosacral foramenectomies, and bilateral lumbar sympathectomies. Despite the surgeries and other procedures, he reported having constant back pain and spent only two hours per day in nonreclining activities. At the time he was admitted to the rehabilitation unit, he was taking analgesic medication for the pain, and sedatives in order to be able to sleep.

In the hospital, his medication immediately was placed on a time-contingent basis and was delivered in a color and taste masking vehicle. By the tenth week following his admission, the medication had been reduced to the masking vehicle only.

During the first four days of his hospitalization, the patient was

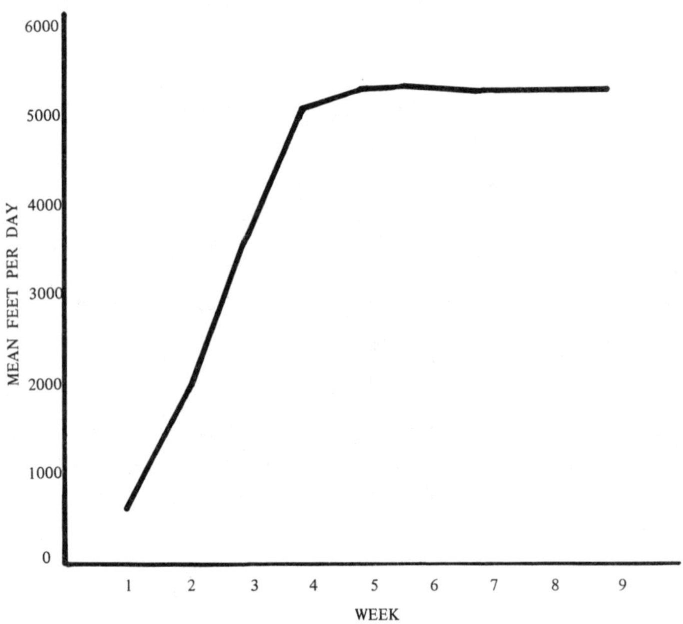

Figure 10-3 Patient's mean daily walking distance by week. From Fordyce, W. E., Fowler, R. S., Lehmann, J. F. and DeLateur, Barbara: Some implications of learning in problems of chronic pain. *J Chronic Dis, 21*:179, 1968.

Reproduced with the permission of the senior author and the *Journal of Chronic Disease*. Copyright 1968, Pergamon Press.

observed on an ambulation program. Then quotas were placed on his walking, which he had to meet in order to receive the reinforcer of rest. These quotas were increased gradually.

Figure 10-3 shows his mean daily walking distance per week. From the first week, he ambulated greater and greater distances until no additional quotas were placed on this behavior.

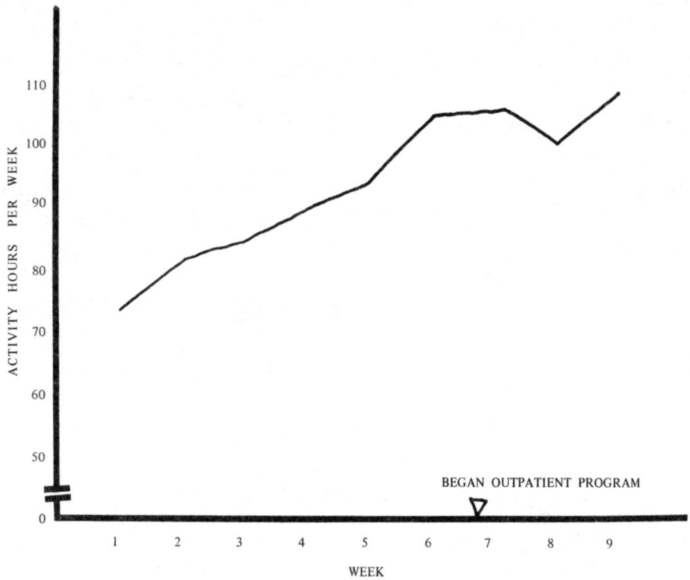

Figure 10-4 Total hours of activity per week. From Fordyce, W. E., Fowler, R. S., Lehmann, J. F. and DeLateur, Barbara: Some implications of learning in problems of chronic pain. *J Chronic Dis, 21*:179, 1968.

Reproduced with the permission of the senior author and the *Journal of Chronic Disease*. Copyright 1968, Pergamon Press.

The patient's general level of activity increased significantly, as can be seen in Figure 10-4, and he began to explore vocational goals as well.

* * * * *

In a research investigation which employed the behavioral

approach with thirty-six patients having chronic pain problems, Fordyce, Fowler, Lehmann, DeLateur, Sand and Trieschmann (1973) obtained success in all cases for the variables of reduced medication intake, increased ambulation distances, and increased general level of activity.

Fordyce and his associates feel that two general implications are supported by the data. First, the diagnostic process in problems of chronic pain must consider the effects of learning. It is not the case that pain originally is produced by operant conditioning, but rather that a great deal of pain behavior occurring subsequent to the initial insult may be accounted for and modified by principles of learning. Pain behavior which is under the control of environmental consequences should not look or sound differently from pain behaviors under the control of organic pathology. Thus, diagnostic processes should examine for relationships between the pain phenomena and both pathogenic and environmental factors. Furthermore, when a pain problem has existed for an extended period of time, the opportunities for learning maladaptive behavior by operant mechanism are increased.

The *second* implication is that the treatment of patients with chronic pain may be advanced by the addition of learning procedures to treatment programs. A team approach is required, and the consistency of improvement among patients so treated supports a conclusion that these methods can make valuable contributions to a patient's well-being in problems of chronic pain.

* * * * *

The procedures employed by Fordyce and his colleagues are not the only ones which can be used in dealing with the pain problems of patients. Hollon (1973) presents a case where a somewhat different approach was taken.

A thirty-two year-old woman had sustained brain damage as a result of a gunshot wound. She became right hemiplegic and dysphasic, with a loss of intellectual functioning. She did possess the potential capability for regaining much of her former physical function and ADL skills, and a rehabilitation program was prescribed for her.

However, the patient soon developed an extreme sensitivity to even minimal pain. All efforts to touch her or manipulate her extremities resulted in wails of anguish and frantic pleas to be left alone. This led to strained relationships between the patient and the staff, who felt that much of her pain was imaginary and that her responses were irrational. Personnel were becoming increasingly frustrated by her while she, in turn, complained bitterly that they were "torturing" her. Her rehabilitation treatment was impossible, and transfer to a custodial institution was being considered.

The psychologist designed a program to increase the patient's tolerance for pain and eliminate her wailing and pleading. Observation of the patient revealed that she was most calm and enthusiastic when talking about her home and children. She also could be calmed by having her describe her discomfort in a quiet, conversational manner. This talking would inhibit the wailing and pleading, and allow the patient to tolerate therapeutic procedures for a very brief periods of time. The talking behavior, therefore, was identified as potentially cooperative, self-help behavior which could be shaped into behavior that would increase the patient's pain tolerance.

The staff was instructed not to attempt to touch the patient nor to move her extremities if there were any indications of wailing or pleading. They were not to try to persuade her to stop wailing nor to permit them to touch her under these conditions. They were to ignore completely the entire class of pain-related behaviors and were, instead, to concentrate on encouraging the patient to talk about her children, her home, and her discomfort. When she did this, the staff was to reinforce her behavior by listening attentively, making interested comments, and praising her efforts to speak with them. Only when she was fully engrossed in the talking behavior were they to attempt manipulation of her limbs or other therapeutic procedures which might result in pain or discomfort.

Within several days after this approach was initiated systematically, there was a marked reduction in the patient's wailing and pleading behavior. Within two weeks, a pattern developed in which she would carry on a rambling but composed conversation, while the therapist manipulated her extremities and obtained her cooperation in carrying out procedures, while praising the patient for her efforts. The patient permitted the therapist to conduct exercises which previously had elicited anguished wails and pleas to be left alone. Rehabilitation now became possible.

A second outcome of the study was the patient's realization that she could exercise some control over her own pain. She came to understand that when she engaged in animated conversation she suffered less. Thus, she initiated talking behavior as a means of coping with her pain. This helped to reduce her fear and give her self-confidence.

An interesting feature of Hollon's investigation was the fact that the patient herself provided the means with which to modify her behavior. The psychologist had observed that when she engaged in conversation about certain topics her behavior was more composed and she seemed able to tolerate pain better, although the patient was unaware of the inhibiting effects her talking had on her undesirable behavior. Then he employed this knowledge to treat the patient. After the patient's pain behaviors began to change, she herself came to realize the relationship between her talking and her tolerance for pain, and used her new awareness in a self-therapeutic manner.

It must not be assumed that all pain behaviors can be viewed as operants or that a learning approach can be used with every patient who exhibits chronic pain. This chapter only presented cases where this was, in fact, true. The most pragmatic approach to a problem of chronic pain would be one which employs both the medical model and the behavioral model in the diagnostic process. Both must be considered, and treatment of the pain problem should be contingent upon the paradigm which appears to be most appropriate. If a definite organic pathology is found and a specific medication, treatment modality or surgical procedure is known to be effective with such pathology, a behavioral approach is, of course, not warranted. On the other hand, if no organic pathology is discovered and no standard medical or surgical procedure proves to be successful, persistence with these methods, or assuming that the patient has an "emotional" problem requiring psychotherapy, would be inefficient and ineffective. In the latter instance, an operant conditioning approach should be considered as the treatment of choice because of its repeatedly demonstrated successfulness.

REFERENCES

Fordyce, W. E.: Pain viewed as learned behavior. In Bonica, J. J. (Ed.): *Advances in Neurology,* Vol. 4. New York, Raven, 1974a.

Fordyce, W. E.: Treating chronic pain by contingency management. In Bonica, J. J. (Ed.): *Advances in Neurology,* Vol. 4. New York, Raven, 1974b.

Fordyce, W. E., Fowler, R. S. and DeLateur, Barbara: An application of behavior modification techniques to a problem of chronic pain. *Behav Res Ther, 6*:105, 1968.

Fordyce, W. E., Fowler, R. S., Lehmann, J. F. and DeLateur, Barbara: Some implications of learning in problems of chronic pain. *J Chronic Dis, 21*:179, 1968.

Fordyce, W. E., Fowler, R. S., Lehmann, J. F., DeLateur, Barbara J., Sand, Patricia L. and Trieschmann, Roberta B.: Operant conditioning in the treatment of chronic pain. *Arch Phys Med Rehabil, 54*:399, 1973.

Hollon, T. H.: Behavior modification in a community hospital rehabilitation unit. *Arch Phys Med Rehabil, 54*:65, 1973.

Sternbach, R. A.: *Pain: A Psychophysiological Analysis.* New York, Academic, 1968.

Ullmann, L. P. and Krasner, L. (Eds): *Case Studies in Behavior Modification.* New York, Holt, Rinehart, Winston, 1965.

SECTION V

BIOFEEDBACK IN REHABILITATION

INTRODUCTION

BIOFEEDBACK MAY BE defined as the utilization of externally displayed representations of physiological activities as cues for the learning of the self-regulation of those activities.

The majority of investigations which have employed biofeedback techniques have been of a fundamental or basic nature, and have not been geared towards therapeutic alleviation of human problems. However, biofeedback is increasingly being used as a therapy modality, most frequently for muscle retraining, eliminating tension and migraine headaches, treating cardiac arrhythmias, eliminating subvocal speech during reading, lowering blood pressure in hypertensive patients, and reducing seizures. The results of such studies, while not always conclusive, are at least encouraging. For information on current research in the field, the interested reader can consult Di Cara, Barber, Kamiya, Miller, Shapiro and Stoyva (1974).

This section focuses on biofeedback as a therapeutic procedure for the problems of the physically disabled. Rehabilitation has been an area for such endeavors only within fairly recent years, but it appears to be a safe conclusion that the future will see an increasing number of efforts in the field. It is important to bear in mind, however, that at present, biofeedback must still be viewed primarily as experimental, and that there is much to be learned before it becomes an integral part of patients' total rehabilitation programs.

Chapter Eleven

THERAPEUTIC APPLICATIONS OF BIOFEEDBACK IN REHABILITATION MEDICINE

BIOFEEDBACK DOES NOT correct or cure any problem. Rather, it provides information regarding activity or performance so that a patient may learn to correct the problems himself by gaining control over his own responses. Thus, biofeedback techniques can be viewed as an adjunct to a patient's own abilities, one that enhances his learning to utilize the capacity which he possesses.

STANDING AND WEIGHT BEARING

Herman (1973, 1974a) and Taylor (1974) have reported on a device known as the Limb Load Monitor (LLM), which is designed to measure and display to the patient the total force applied to his lower extremity while standing and ambulating.

The degree and the rate of change of load are detected by a flexible force transducer, in the form of an insole fitted within the patient's shoe. The transducer is wired to a small electronics package which contains the auditory display apparatus and the batteries, and is worn on the patient's belt. The transducer itself consists of foam rubber material sandwiched between layers of copper mylar laminate. It exhibits a capacitance change when force is applied to it. The capacitance change produces a frequency shift of the oscillator in the electronics package, and this shift is converted to a voltage which is used to alter the pitch of an audible tone following its comparison with a predetermined value.

A switch on the device permits three functional modes of display.

Mode 1: As the load increases to the desired level, the frequency of the tone signal decreases to an imperceptible range.

Mode 2: The frequency of the signal is initiated, and increases with loads at or above the desired level.

Mode 3: Utilizing both of the other modes, no auditory signal is perceived between the termination of Mode 1 and the initiation of Mode 2. In other words, no auditory signal is perceived about a preselected null point. The "off" response can be adjusted about the null point or desired loading level.

Reinforcement is achieved by the detection of the immediate disappearance of the signal as in Mode 1, the onset of the signal as in Mode 2, or the lack of feedback between the two signals as in Mode 3.

Twelve patients having either right or left hemiplegia, who had achieved optimal recovery through a rehabilitation therapy program, and who had been disabled for two-and one-half years, completed an initial training program with the LLM. The patients were between thirty and sixty years of age, and their disabilities included varying extents of sensory and motor involvement. All of the patients required some kind of assistive device during ambulation.

Prior to training with the LLM, each patient's weight-bearing pattern was determined during quiet stance. The patients stood on the force plates of a walkway which measured the vertical force under the affected extremity. An additional clinical assessment was made of each patient's ability to perform independent synergy patterns. Sensory disturbances, spasticity, and the use of assistive devices were noted and recorded.

During training the patients were seen once or twice per week for thirty-minute sessions. At the start of each session the patient's body weight was measured, he was equipped with an LLM, and the device was calibrated for 50 percent of his body weight. A training session consisted of an initial assessment of standing performance and a practice period of twenty minutes duration. The practice period involved one minute of standing and one minute of resting, with feedback elicited periodically, i.e. each one-minute period, alternate periods, every third period, etc., depending upon the patient's level of performance. The auditory feedback signal indicated to the patient the magnitude of an error in loading.

Training sessions also were conducted at home. These sessions were of thirty minutes in length, consisting of one minute standing periods utilizing feedback with brief rest intervals between trials. A family member of the patient conducted the home training.

As a final assessment procedure, the patient stood on the force plates for two minutes without feedback. If he met the criterion for equal weight-bearing, i.e. 10 percent or less load difference between the lower extremities, he was given four slight pushes, one from each side. If he was able to resume his position after each push, the feedback training was terminated.

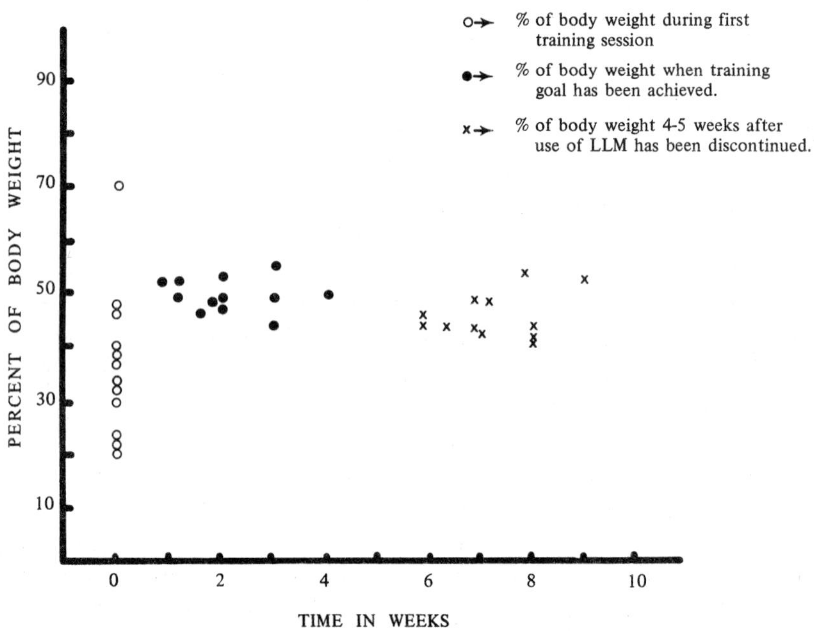

Figure 11-1 Percent of body weight maintained on hemiparetic limb. From Herman, R.: *Biofeedback*. Paper presented at the Regional Training Session on Cerebral Palsy, Harrisburg, 1974.

Reproduced with the permission of the author.

Following conclusion of the training program, a follow-up of each patient was conducted once per week for one month. Ten of the subjects were evaluated after one month and again after six months. At these times, their weight-bearing pattern was determined as before, and their functional status was reevaluated.

The results of this investigation are presented in Figure 11-1. It can be seen that only two of the twelve subjects were able to maintain an even balance of weight prior to being trained with the LLM. Four of the patients required more than two weeks to achieve an even standing load, three needed three weeks, and one took four weeks. By the fourth week, all subjects were maintaining good weight balance.

One month after the termination of the study, three patients were found to exhibit a decline in loading and weight-bearing on the affected lower extremity ranging between 33 percent and 43

Patient	Sex	Age	Funct. Diagnosis	Treatment With Limb Load Monitor					
				Initial Loading Status % Body Wt.	Discharge Loading Status % Body Wt.	Initial Assistive Device	Final Assistive Device	No. of Treatment Sessions	Mean Treatment Time (in Min.)
1	F	38	Left Hemi.	.42	.77	Parallel Bars	Parallel Bars	9	20
2	F	62	Left Hemi.	.46	.46	Parallel Bars	Parallel Bars	4	25
3	M	18	Left Hemi.	.34	.69	Quad Cane	Quad Cane	1	25
4	M	45	Left Hemi.	.50	.85	Paral. Bars Cane	Paral. Bars Cane	3	60
5	M	40	Left Hemi.	.29	.51	Parallel Bars	Cane	4	30
6	M	24	Left Limb Paresis & Fem. Fract.	.79	.69	Cane	Crutches	10	60
7	F	64	Left Hemi.	.23	.50	Cane	Cane	4	35
8	M	37	Left Hemi.	.17	.92	Parallel Bars	Cane	8	25
9	M	50	R. & L. Hemi.	.39	.95	Parallel Bars	Parallel Bars	10	60

Table 11-I Initial and post-treatment status of nine patients receiving therapy with the Limb Load Monitor. From Herman, R.: *Biofeedback.* Paper presented at the Regional Training Session on Cerebral Palsy, Harrisburg, 1974. Reproduced with the permission of the author.

percent of body weight. These patients had taken longer than two weeks to gain control of standing and two of them had sensory disturbances. Six months later there were no changes observed in their status.

The functional reevaluations which were conducted during the follow-up sessions indicated increasing independence in standing activities for the majority of the subjects, with less reliance on assistive aids during ambulation. It was apparent that the patients used the LLM to gain control over ambulation once postural control had been achieved.

A second study, involving ten additional patients using the LLM, has been conducted. Table 11-I presents the data for the nine patients who completed the training program. Seven of the patients increased limb loading and two progressed to a less supportive assistive device. These results were achieved within a brief number of sessions. The mean session duration was forty minutes.

The therapists who worked with the subjects felt that the LLM was both useful and needed in clinical treatment, and nearly all of the patients stated that the device helped them to "sense" the load on the involved extremity.

* * * * *

Herman and his associates (Herman, 1973) have developed a modified standing table which provides feedback to the patient regarding improper trunk, hip and/or knee alignment, and asymmetrical loading of the lower extremities. The table also increases the balance performance and standing tolerance of patients with sensorimotor deficits.

A pressure detection system informs both the patient and the therapist of abnormal postural movements, including undue loading of either lower extremity, knee and hip flexion, or shifting of the trunk in an anterior/posterior direction. The occurrence of any of these movements activates both a visual and an auditory signal, providing a sensory display of one or more errors in body position.

Two foot mats with mat switches are positioned on the floor of the unit so that the patient can place his feet evenly on each mat. Two ribbon switches, one each for the knee and the back, are located under the cushion pads along the top portion of the knee rest and the back rest. These are energized whenever the patient flexes his knees or leans posteriorly. The circuitry for the operation of the switches and the sensory display signals are contained in a control box.

The patient is positioned inside the standing table with the knee pad and the back rest individually adjusted. When the patient's feet are weight-bearing and correctly placed on the foot mats, left and right foot lights are on. The knee and back indicator lights are off when the patient is standing correctly, i.e. neither leaning posteriorly nor resting his knees on the knee board.

When the patient shifts his body weight or raises either foot, the appropriate light is shut off and an audible buzzer is activated. When the patient leans back or flexes his knees, the buzzer sounds, and the appropriate light signal is triggered. The desired positions and forces for each patient can be adjusted so that responses are progressively shaped to their final, desired form.

While extensive data are not available yet from studies conducted with this apparatus, Herman has reported that it "has been found to be quite useful in attaining postural and equilibrium control in patients with both musculoskeletal (e.g. rheumatoid arthritis and amputations) and neurological (e.g. hemiplegia) disorders."

According to Herman, neural control of posture can be preprogrammed at the supraspinal level. When there are neurosensory disturbances there often follows a rearrangement of the supraspinal command centers. These changes interfere with the spatiotemporal organization of motor behaviors, and thus lead to disturbances of postural control. The result of this is an inability of the central nervous system to recalibrate load or force sensed by the lower extremities during performance into precise functioning. Recalibration of function may, in fact, even decay when response feedback no longer is available.

The sensory aids, such as the Limb Load Monitor and the modified standing table, which have been described, provide relevant, precise and consistent sensory information of dynamic performance. This information is delivered to the patient through intact sensory channels without temporal delay, thus making the patient continually aware of the magnitude and direction of success or error of performance. Reinforcement, attentiveness, and motivation, therefore, are an integral part of the therapy program on a response-contingent basis, which typically is not the case with traditional therapist-patient interactions.

The Limb Load Monitor provides precise monitoring of partial weight-bearing, an orderly progression in control of incremental weight-bearing and sustained maximal weight-bearing, and regulates postural and equilibrium responses.

If ambulation is viewed as a series of postural adjustments, by effecting optimal calibration of forces and position when the subject is upright, then the modified standing table provides essential prerequisites for walking.

These devices, in addition to providing patients with the necessary awareness of their performance for improvement, free the therapist from having to remain by the patient's side as he performs, provide more precise measures and reinforcement than are possible in traditional therapeutic approaches, and provide therapeutic practice for longer time periods than can be implemented by a therapist alone.

AMBULATION

The basic biofeedback principle of providing patients with an awareness of their performance has been applied in the area of locomotive behavior (Craik, Wannstedt and Hesson, 1974; Herman, 1974b; Taylor, 1974).

The Step Length Monitor (SLM) is an apparatus which supplies the patient with feedback of step length symmetry while it simultaneously gives the therapist an accurate and objective measure of performance.

The SLM consists of a small, battery-operated control box and two plug-in sensor elements. The sensors are mounted on the patient's lower extremities, just above the medial malleolus on each ankle, and are affixed with Velcro® straps. The distance between the sensors is measured by transmitting a short burst of .40 Khz ultrasonic energy at a rate of 500 times per second from one sensor which is received by the other and measuring the elapsed time. The time elapsed between emission of the energy and its reception is a direct measure of the separation of the two sensor elements and, thus, of ankle separation. The time interval controls the pitch of an audible signal emitted from a loudspeaker to display the measured ankle distance.

The SLM, therefore, provides a continuous measure of foot separation while a patient ambulates. It is the difference between this measure and a predetermined distance which is displayed as the tone. A switch on the apparatus makes it possible to have the tone sound either for step lengths which are longer or shorter than the predetermined value. The device also is connected to a pen and ink recorder which provides an immediate readout of the patient's gait velocity in addition to step length. The SLM has a reliable range of measurement of from 2 to 24 inches.

Both hemiplegic patients and normal subjects have been tested with the SLM. All six of the hemiplegics exhibited asymmetry in temporal and spatial gait variables.

For the normal subjects, when data has been collected on their usual step length, the device was set arbitrarily to provide feedback at a different step length. These subjects were able to achieve and maintain the new, required step length after only a few steps.

With the hemiplegic patients, the level of the feedback display was set at approximately one-half of their usual stride length, as was determined prior to training. This was found to be the most functional method of achieving symmetry of step length without a loss of velocity or a reduction of safety during walking. Once a patient responded satisfactorily, the step length gradually was increased during the subsequent training sessions.

It was found that all of the hemiplegic patients approached the desired symmetry of step length within the initial session, although they required more time to do so than did the normal subjects. The ratio of the longer step to the shorter step ranged from 1.2 to 2.2 inches at baseline, and from 1.2 to 1.5 when the auditory feedback was employed.

The significance of the Step Length Monitor lies in its capacity to provide both the patient and the therapist with immediate feedback of locomotor performance on a continuous basis during ambulation. This enables the patient to practice independently, and to practice his gait pattern during times when he is not in the physical therapy area, but is on his ward or floor, or in his home. Since the feedback is constant, this apparatus should also reduce the time necessary for rehabilitation.

The SLM, like the Limb Load Monitor and the modified standing table, previously described in this chapter, also permits the therapist to use her time more efficiently with the patient.

* * * * *

Wooldridge (1974) has developed a biofeedback system to correct abnormal knee positions during ambulation in children with cerebral palsy. A potentiometer is connected to two metal arms which serve as a goniometer. Plastic cuffs with Velcro® fasteners are attached to each arm and hold the goniometer in place at the knee joint. The position of the knee joint is translated into an audible tone whose frequency varies in direct proportion with the joint position. Auditory information can be provided throughout the entire range of joint motion, at any point in the range, or can be omitted at any point in the range. The electronics package that converts the joint motion into the auditory signal can be worn on the patient's belt. During training sessions, a stop watch records elapsed time, and a step counter records the number of strides and errors made by the patient.

A six-year-old boy, with mild-moderate spastic diplegia was ambulating with a parallel pusher, with his hips and knees flexed, and his heels barely touching the ground. The initial contact which his foot made with the floor was with his forefoot. Measurement of range of movement in his lower extremities showed that, passively, his knees barely extended to zero degrees. The dynamic range of knee flexion and extension of the child's right leg was determined to be between 38 and 52 degrees during ambulation.

Positive feedback, in the form of the auditory tone, was given to the patient when he extended his right knee in stance to 35 degrees. Each trial consisted of ambulating a distance of 100 feet, during which the feedback condition was operative. Records were kept of the number of strides which the child took with the right foot, the number of times the goal was achieved, and the total time of each trial.

Sixteen training sessions were conducted. At the beginning of the training, each time the patient's right knee extended past 35 degrees he received the auditory feedback. On the first day, the percent achievement of the desired goal averaged 58 percent over all trials. Within five sessions, the predetermined performance goal of 75 percent success rate was achieved. The feedback was withdrawn during the sixth session, and the patient's success rate declined to 31 percent. Reinstatement of the feedback at a thirty-degree extension criterion resulted in 83 percent success. It decreased, subsequently, but after three feedback sessions it rose to 83 percent again. The feedback condition was removed once more, and the patient's success rate dropped to 15 percent.

Within a brief period of time, the biofeedback training had enabled the patient to alter his knee extension pattern during ambulation, which his physical therapist had been unable to achieve in five months of training. However, while the child was able to perform well under conditions of reinforcement, each time the reinforcement condition was withdrawn, his performance declined markedly. In addition, there was little generalization from the training sessions to daily activity. One must conclude, therefore, that this child's motor pattern was not basically changed.

* * * * *

Greater success was achieved with an eight-year-old boy diagnosed as having spastic diplegia. He had undergone surgery to divide the iliopsoas, and release the hip adductors and the proximal hamstring muscles. Two years postsurgery he still ambulated with his trunk flexed forward and his crutches approximately 2 feet in front of him. His heel cords were tight, and his knees went into recurvatum.

A biofeedback program was designed to give the child better knee control and to prevent the recurvatum that occurred with each step he took. Since the left lower extremity was the weaker one, it was selected for training. The auditory tone was set to activate from 10 degrees to hyperextension. The general program consisted of individual balancing and gait training, and additional use of the joint position trainer for approximately thirty minutes in the child's school room during a free activity period.

The program began with five 2-minute trials of standing balance while the child worked at a puzzle or a game at a table. Then this was changed to one-minute sessions of free-standing balance, while the therapist attempted to disturb the child's equilibrium. The patient learned to control his posture within one session.

Ambulation training consisted of five trials in the school corridor or on the pavement outdoors, in which 50 strides were made with the left foot. Data were collected on errors and elapsed time for each 50 strides.

Prior to training, the patient made an error at each of the 50 steps. His performance time was one minute and thirty-four seconds. During the first biofeedback session he made 24 errors for the 50 strides. On the second day of training he ambulated 50 steps with only one error, but required four minutes and forty-eight seconds to do so. By the tenth day of the feedback condition, the patient was averaging three errors per 50 steps, and was taking two minutes and nine seconds to walk the distance. The feedback was withdrawn during the next session but he maintained his rate of ambulation and made only three errors over five trials. After one week of no training, the patient was tested in his home without feedback. He was requiring three minutes and twenty seconds to walk 50 steps, but made no errors. In addition, there were improvements in foot alignment and swing without loss of stride length. The child became able to modify his gait at will, although he reverted to his former pattern when in a hurry.

This second case presents a rather dramatic example of the success of biofeedback. Not only was the child able to correct his knee position during ambulation while in training in the hospital, but was able to maintain his performance at home. The fact that when he was hurried he reverted to his pretraining gait pattern may be an indication of extinction. This problem may be correctable with additional training where feedback is given on an intermittent rather than a continuous basis, as in a reinforcement schedule, and under conditions where the child must hurry, rather than being permitted unlimited time to complete the task.

ELECTROMYOGRAPHIC FEEDBACK AS THERAPY

Electromyography (EMG) is the diagnostic technique which

deals with the detection, recording, and interpretation of the electrical voltages generated by skeletal muscle (Ince, 1974). These electrical potentials are displayed auditorily and/or visually in the study of muscle and nerve physiology. Within recent years, the EMG has been found to be a useful therapeutic modality when employed in feedback training (Blanchard and Young, 1974).

Brudny, Korein, Friedmann, Grynbaum, Weinstein and Frankel (1974) treated sixty-three patients having a wide variety of clinical disorders over a two-year period using audiovisual displays of EMG.

The treatment population included six patients with peripheral nerve injuries, two patients with quadriparesis, eighteen patients with hemiparesis, twenty-four with spasmodic torticollis, four with hemifacial spasms, seven dystonic patients and two patients having muscle atrophy secondary to injury or disease. The age range of the patients was from thirteen to eighty-one years, and the duration of illness varied between nine months and thirty-five years. Each patient was examined by a neurologist and a physiatrist prior to participation in the study, and each was informed that he might learn better control of functionally defective muscles, but that a cure was not being offered.

Prior to treatment, baseline measures were obtained of peripheral blood flow, EEG, EMG, and integrated EMG up to four muscles. The EMG recordings were made with the muscles at rest and also during maximal voluntary or involuntary activity. All of the recordings were repeated after eight to twelve weeks of therapy. Videotape recordings of the degree of functional deficiency of movement disorder were made before therapy was initiated.

Only surface electrodes were employed. The EMG signal was amplified, rectified and integrated by a digital computer which permitted simultaneous integration of signals from two muscles in microvolt-seconds. A digital print-out provided continuous data on the electrical activity of the two muscles under study. An oscilloscope visually displayed the integrated muscle potentials. The tracing continually exhibited the degree and rate of muscle contractions immediately upon their occurrence. An auditory display presented changes in EMG activity either by proportional changes in the intensity of the sound, or by a signal which was emitted after a correct response.

Prior to initiating the biofeedback treatment, the deficient motor activity of each patient was analyzed and therapeutic goals were determined. These included reaching, grasping, pulling, or control of involuntary muscle movement, such as spasmodic or spastic activity. The desired motor behavior then was subdivided into a series of simple tasks performed by the prime movers, the agonists, and therapy was directed towards the learning of voluntary control over those muscles. The synergists and antagonist muscles then were treated similarly. The patients' initial efforts were directed towards volitional changes of the audiovisual displays of the integrated EMG activity and not towards an actual motor task, although this often occurred.

The desired responses of the patients were achieved through a shaping process, using both the auditory and visual displays of performance. The auditory signal provided reinforcement for successful spatial and temporal responding on a task. The patients' volitional muscle responses were displayed visually against an arbitrary voltage line which represented the therapeutic goals, and which gradually was modified by the therapist in the desired direction, over several sessions. As the patients' muscle responses more closely approximated the designated therapy goal, the visual feedback was withdrawn. The auditory feedback was continued concomitant with direct visual observation of the involved body part by the patient.

When inhibition or suppression of undesired, involuntary antagonistic muscle activity was required, feedback from the activity of two muscles, agonist and antagonist, was given simultaneously. The activity of these muscles was displayed either through the two different sensory channels, or both were shown through the visual modality alone, or only one was displayed auditorily.

As the functional components of a desired task returned, and the speed and accuracy of performance improved, the biofeedback was withdrawn gradually. Treatment sessions were spaced further apart and gradually were discontinued as a patient became able to carry out adequate functional movement repeatedly without feedback.

The therapeutic sessions were conducted three to five times per week. Each session was of approximately thirty to forty-five minutes long, with several rest periods scheduled during each session.

The results of the biofeedback therapy were evaluated clinically, in terms of functional gains, following eight to twelve weeks of treatment.

Of the fifteen hemiparetic patients with whom treatment was directed at improved upper extremity function, assistive capacity and prehension were established in eleven cases. Two patients obtained relief from spasticity, and two others showed no changes.

Retraining of the lower extremities was attempted with three hemiparetic patients. One of the patients, who gained control of ankle dorsiflexion, showed significant generalization during ambulation. The other two did not make such gains.

Prior to biofeedback training, only three of the patients with spasmodic torticollis were able to maintain their head in a neutral position voluntarily, and then only for a few minutes. Following the EMG feedback sessions, fourteen of these patients could maintain a neutral neck position for hours and longer. Nine were able to do so for from two to thirty minutes, and one patient, while able to maintain a neutral position of his head for hours, could do so only with biofeedback.

Among the dystonic patients, improvement was observed in only two cases who previously had undergone cryothalamectomies. Complaints were limited to one or two muscles in these patients.

The upper extremities were treated in the quadriparetic patients, both of whom had lesions at the C_5—C_6 level of the spinal cord. Both patients became able to achieve prehension ability through voluntary control of spasticity and wrist tenodesis activity after not having this ability for eighteen months and two years, respectively.

Two of the four patients having facial spasms were able to learn satisfactory control over the involuntary muscle activity. They were able to return to work with only occasional recurrence of the problem.

Both patients with severe secondary quadriceps muscle atrophy achieved control of voluntary contractions for increase of muscle bulk and strength, and as a result, both became ambulatory.

The patients who were recovering from peripheral nerve injuries learned to use their transferred wrist flexor tendons for wrist extension within only two 30-minute sessions.

These results demonstrate the feasibility and utility of biofeedback as a therapeutic modality in cases of loss or impairment of neuromotor control. Brudny and his colleagues propose the following hypothesis to account for the learned control.

During the feedback therapy, the audiovisual signals which indicate muscle activity appear to have special matching characteristics with regard to information pertaining to the degree and rate of muscle contraction. Normally, this information is provided by the proprioceptive system. The audiovisual sensory feedback from muscle activity is a substitution for, or augmentation of, proprioceptive feedback, in the relearning of patterned movements. When delivered with the appropriate degree of modulation through intact sensory channels, and translated by the neural mechanism aided by the plasticity of the brain, auditory and visual signals apparently are able to stimulate the sensorimotor corticothalamic loops and subcortical systems in a manner which produces a selective pattern of motor outflow (Brudny, et al., 1974). This phenomenon, which initially occurs at random, becomes more consistent through operant conditioning training so that a meaningful patterned movement is retained. This suggests that the biofeedback results in new sensorimotor integration.

Since, after the onset of a disability, there may be much of a previously learned pattern of movement still intact within the central nervous system, many repetitions of movement are not necessary for relearning to take place. Thus, return of movement can occur rapidly. However, it appears to be crucial that the modality which is used as a substitute possesses characteristics which are related directly to the sensory component which is missing. The information on the temporal and spatial changes in the muscle is most important so that this information eventually can be incorporated into the relearned neural nets, subserving voluntary movement, and be retained (Brudny et al., 1974). The audiovisual displays of integrated EMG appear to be just such a substitute modality, capable of providing or augmenting the missing information accurately and promptly, which is essential for the relearning of movement patterns.

The Treatment of Spasmodic Torticollis

Torticollis is a spasmodic contraction of the neck muscles, primarily those supplied by the spinal accessory nerve. The head is drawn to one side and usually rotated, often causing severe discomfort as well as embarrassment. In addition, the disorder can produce a difficulty or inability to perform certain tasks, particularly those requiring fine visual-motor coordination. Thus, the general consequences of torticollis may be quite disabling. The etiology of the disorder is questionable and chemotherapeutic and surgical treatment procedures have had only limited success.

Cleeland (1973) employed a combination of EMG feedback and electric shock in his treatment of nine patients with torticollis and one with retrocollis, where the head is drawn backward.

Surface electrodes were placed near the anterior border, and just above the clavicular attachment of the right and left sternocleidomastoid muscles. EMG activity was recorded, as were the other stimuli used in the study, i.e. electric shock and auditory EMG feedback display. The EMG activity was amplified and fed into a voltage-controlled oscillator which controlled a tone that varied in pitch proportionate to the changing EMG signals. The tone was presented through an audio amplifier and a speaker.

Amplified EMG activity also was fed to an adjustable Schmitt trigger, the output of which could activate a cutaneous electric shock. A stimulator with a step-up isolation transformer delivered current to two plate electrodes attached to the patient's first and second fingers. Pulse trains of ten per second, with a pulse duration of 10 milliseconds, were employed. The amount of current per pulse varied between two and four milliamperes. The shock remained on as long as the threshhold voltage of the Schmitt trigger was exceeded.

The patient heard the auditory display of EMG signals through a speaker in the experimental room. The pitch change of the feedback proportional to the EMG varied between 200 and 1500 Hz. The range was adjusted individually proportional to the amplitude of each patient's spasm. Spasms were recorded on an electric counter controlled by the Schmitt trigger.

In the experimental procedure, each patient received continuous, on-line information regarding the relative EMG activity in the involved muscles. Shock was delivered to the finger electrodes upon an initial increase in EMG amplitude. That is, the shock was initiated at the onset of a spasm. The shock remained on as long as the spasm continued.

	Age	*Sex*	*Symptom duration*	*Sessions*	*Initial spasm frequency/ 5 minutes*	*Final spasm frequency/ 5 minutes*	*Shock effect*	*Initial improvement*	*Follow-up improvement (duration)*
Case 1	15	M	4 months	16	44	3	+	++	++ (18 months)
Case 2	25	F	60 months	6	21	6	+	+	+ (40 months)
Case 3	64	M	36 months	23	188	168	0	0	0 (17 months)
Case 4	50	F	24 months	10	40	1	+	+	+ (18 months)
Case 5	28	M	9 months	8	75	46	+	+	Lost to follow-up
Case 6*	54	F	36 months	8	40	0	+	++	+ (17 months)
Case 7	18	F	2 months	15	11	0	+	++	++ (24 months)
Case 8	54	F	10 months	10	54	11	+	+	0 (20 months)
Case 9	43	F	7 months	8	34	8	0	+	0 (5 months)
Case 10	32	M	6 months	8	28	5	+	++	++ (1 month)

*Retrocollis.

Table 11-II Data for nine patients with torticollis and one with retrocollis. From Cleeland, C. S.: Behavioral technics in the modification of spasmodic torticollis. *Neurology 23*:1241, 1973.

Reproduced with the permission of the author and *Neurology, 23*:1243, Copyright: The New York Times Media Company, Inc.

Table 11-II presents the data for the ten patients involved in the study. In the table, "++" indicates marked improvement, the patient exhibiting no spasmodic activity on follow-up EMG recordings and reporting no spasmodic activity outside of the laboratory. The "+" notation means that there was moderate improvement, the patient showing reduced spasm frequency on follow-up EMG recordings, having significantly reduced head deviation and spasmodic activity as judged by at least two neurologists, and reporting consistent reduction of head deviation and spasm outside of the laboratory. Patients who did not meet all of the criteria for moderate improvement are designated in the table by "O," signifying minimal or no improvement.

It is clear, from inspection of the table, that four patients showed initial marked improvement and three maintained this improvement over the follow-up period, which varied from one to twenty-four months post-treatment. Moderate improvement was observed initially in five patients, three of them remaining improved during a seventeen to forty month follow-up period. One patient did not exhibit any initial improvement, nor was improvement found to have occurred seventeen months later. Two of the patients who had shown an initial moderate improvement had their responses return to pretreatment baseline level within five and twenty months, respectively, post-treatment. In sum, 60 percent of all cases demonstrated moderate or marked improvement in their condition.

Trials using EMG feedback plus electric shock were compared with trials during which feedback alone was used for all of the patients. In eight of the ten patients, feedback plus shock trials resulted in a lower frequency of spasms than did trials in which only feedback was employed during more than half of the sessions when shock was administered. Two patients exhibited little or no further reduction of spasms with the addition of shock.

The effects of EMG-triggered shock alone were studied in one patient. Shock trials were presented randomly during all sessions, together with trials of feedback plus shock, and trials of feedback alone. The shock-feedback trials resulted in significantly fewer spasms than the trials using only shock, and fewer spasms than the trials of feedback alone, although this latter finding was not statistically significant.

There are several possible explanations for the results obtained in this investigation. Spasmodic torticollis is manifested as both spasmodic activity and excessive background EMG activity, usually in one sternocleidomastoid muscle, but frequently generalizing to other muscle groups. Electric shock has been found to reduce the frequency of tics in various muscle groups when the shock was made contingent upon tics (Yates, 1958), and EMG feedback has been demonstrated as successful in reducing muscle tension in patients with neck injuries (Jacobs and Felton, 1969). Thus, the combination of shock and feedback may be the most effective way of treating a spasm disorder.

Cleeland speculated that the effects obtained through the use of shock may be attributable to an escape or avoidance conditioning model, but he also pointed out that the shock may have reduced the frequency of spasms on a reflexive basis, since such has been demonstrated in torticollis (Podivinsky, 1969). He feels, however, that it may at least partially be assumed that slight increases in sternocleidomastoid activity, and thus in the feedback signal, did become a conditioned stimulus for the occurrence of both spasm and shock. This assumption appears particularly tenable in light of the fact that many of the patients involved in the study reported that the EMG feedback gave them an "image" of sternocleidomastoid activity which they did not have before. It was this new proprioception which enabled them voluntarily to relax the muscles.

It may have been the case that the shock did serve as a punisher for undesirable EMG activity, hence the situation may be described as one of escape and avoidance conditioning. This, then, either facilitated the learning of correct EMG responses, or the learning of EMG activity through biofeedback enhanced the escape and avoidance learning. Thus, it would appear that both are necessary for effective muscle control.

* * * * *

Brudny, Grynbaum and Korein (1974), however, achieved success in treating spasmodic torticollis through the use of EMG feedback alone.

Seven men and two women, aged twenty to fifty-eight years, were seen in treatment. The duration of their disability varied between nine months and fifteen years. Six of the patients had torticollis with the chin pointing to the left, and three with the chin pointing to the right. In addition, five of the patients had scoliosis and four exhibited signs of torsion dystonia.

EMG signals, detected by surface electrodes on the sternocleidomastoid muscles, were amplified, filtered, rectified and integrated. The integration permitted adequate quantification of changing EMG signals at any time. The changes were displayed both visually and auditorily.

The visual display consisted of a dial pointer on a calibrated scale which showed an arbitrary number correlated to the magnitude of integrated EMG signals at any given time. The auditory feedback was a rising and falling intensity of sound by means of a changing click rate approximately proportional to the integrated EMG activity.

The therapeutic goals were defined as a volitional decrease of spasm in the spasmodic muscle and a volitional increase of contraction and strength in the contralateral muscle.

Learning to volitionally change the levels of the EMG feedback display resulted in learning control of muscle activity, since the former was an instant reflection of changes in the latter. The patients rapidly came to understand the relationship between muscle contraction and relaxation and the corresponding changes in the feedback displays.

The treatment sessions were of thirty to sixty minutes duration, and were conducted from three to five times per week over a mean period fo ten weeks. Once a patient became able to maintain a neutral neck position throughout a session, the sessions were spaced farther apart and eventually were discontinued. The patients were given a home program of daily maximal isometric contractions of the previously atrophied contralateral muscle, and were instructed to continue this indefinitely and to use the exercise whenever a spasm recurred.

The stated goals of the treatment program gradually were achieved, and the patients were required to perform better as the study progressed. It was found that the neck usually could be kept in a neutral position volitionally when the values of the integrated EMG signals became equal over the muscles of both sides of the neck.

Seven of the nine patients became able to overcome spasms voluntarily without the need of biofeedback, and all but two continued or resumed their employment. Table 11-III shows the degree of self-control of each patient during therapy and without feedback after therapy.

Brudny and his associates feel that the brain's plasticity may permit the integration of external sensory signals which substitute for impaired "normal" internal sensory processing mechanisms delivered through intact sensory organs; this in turn may produce a reestablishment of voluntary control over muscle activity. Initially the patient responds to a stimulus whose nature has been altered, but while volitionally changing his neck position he also is learning to discriminate other sensory cues from in-

Case no.	Duration of neutral neck position with feedback during therapy	Duration of neutral neck position without feedback following therapy	Ability to resume the disturbed neutral position, volitionally and without feedback	Periodic reinforcement
1	Indefinite	Months	Yes	No
2	Indefinite	Months	Yes	No
3	Indefinite	Hours	Yes	No*
4	Indefinite	Months	Yes	No
5	30 minutes	2-5 minutes	At times only	Yes
6	Indefinite	Hours	Yes	No*
7	Indefinite	5-10 minutes	No	Yes
8	Indefinite	Hours	Yes	No
9	Hours	2-5 minutes	Yes	Yes

*Occasional spasmodic episodes were reported to occur at times in relation to emotional stress or fatigue.

Table 11-III Degree of volitional control of neutral neck position following therapy. From Brudny, J., Grynbaum, B. B. and Korein, J.: Spasmodic torticollis: Treatment by feedback display of the EMG. *Arch Phys Med Rehabil,* 55:403, 1974.

Reproduced with the permission of the senior author and the *Archives of Physical Medicine and Rehabilitation.*

tact sensory modalities and may retain these patterns for correct performance when the feedback displays no longer are present.

The fact that treatment required several weeks should not be considered as contraindicatory to using biofeedback therapeutically. In view of the considerable length of time during which many of the patients had experienced their disorders, treatment of several weeks or months duration can be considered as relatively brief. However, in terms of absolute time and the large number of hours which a clinician (psychologist, physician, etc.) must spend with each patient, it does appear to be a somewhat lengthy and effortful procedure. If, as is hoped by investigators in the field, biofeedback is to become a routine part of the general armamentarium of rehabilitation techniques, some modifications will have to be made so that success can be achieved more rapidly and with less constant staff commitment.

BIOFEEDBACK AND THE LEARNED CONTROL OF BLOOD PRESSURE

There have been a number of studies conducted during the past few years which have demonstrated that man can learn to control certain autonomic functions. Changes in heart rate and blood pressure usually have been slight, and the question has been raised as to whether the autonomic nervous system has been conditioned directly or whether other processes, such as skeletal muscle mediation or cognition are responsible for the obtained results.

Research done with rats paralyzed by curare has shown that skeletal muscle activity probably is not involved in the process (Di Cara and Miller, 1969), but there have been few such studies conducted which involve human subjects.

Pickering, Brucker, Dworkin and Miller (1975) performed a series of experiments to determine whether or not paralyzed humans can learn to modify their blood pressure.

The subjects were eight patients with severe, generalized paralysis of the body, including all four extremities. Four of the patients were postpoliomyelitis quadriplegics, and four patients were paralyzed as the result of muscular dystrophy. All of the subjects had respiratory insufficiency and required mechanical respiratory assistance. With the exception of one patient with fascioscapulohumeral muscular dystrophy affecting only certain muscle groups, the paralysis was nearly complete in all of the subjects, facial and throat muscle activity and slight hand movements being the only ones possible.

All subjects were seen experimentally while they were in their wheelchairs and breathing with their usual respiratory aids. Diastolic blood pressure was recorded continuously, using a servo-controlled sphygmomanometer actuated by Korotkoff sound intensity. The pressure in the cuff of the sphygmomanometer was measured by a transducer and recorded on a Grass polygraph. The amplified and integrated Korotkoff sound also was recorded. The ECG was obtained from precordial electrodes and the EMG was measured from skin electrodes placed under the chin. Respiration was recorded from a mercury-in-rubber strain gauge attached to the chest. All measures were recorded on the polygraph.

The output of the diastolic pressure channel drove a slave channel on the polygraph, for adjustment of the criterion level of pressure at which the patient received feedback. The criterion level corresponded to a fixed voltage from the output jack of this channel, and could be changed in either direction. The output from the channel was passed through a Schmitt trigger to a logic circuit, which activated a pleasant-sounding tone whenever the patient's diastolic pressure was above or below criterion, depending upon the direction in which he was attempting to change his blood pressure. The outputs from the EMG and respiration channels also were fed to the Schmitt trigger and the logic unit so that excess activity in either channel prevented the tone from sounding.

A print-out counter presented the average diastolic blood pressure every fifteen seconds,as well as heart rate, and percentage time of each fifteen-second period during which the criterion level was reached.

All subjects were seen individually. The recording apparatus was separated from the subjects by a screen. After a subject had been connected to the apparatus, and the diastolic monitor had been set to track diastolic blood pressure accurately, the subject was told that he was going to be learning to try and change his blood pressure. He was not told in which direction the changes should occur. The subject was informed that the way to do this was to concentrate on keeping the tone on for as long as he could, but not to alter his breathing in any way or to try and tense his muscles.

Each experimental session consisted of ten 2-minute recordings. The first and the last recordings were used as baseline measures, during which the subject was instructed not to try and change his blood pressure. The tone was not operative during these times. Thus, there were eight trials of training, during which the subject attempted to maintain the tone. During the first five sessions, the full two-minute trial period was used for this training. For the remaining sessions, the first 30 seconds of each trial was employed as a baseline period only. There was a three-minute rest interval between trials. Between alternate trials, blood pressure calibrations were performed. Each session was of approximately sixty minutes duration. All subjects were seen for a minimum of five sessions, and the mean interval between sessions was six days.

A questionnaire was administered to each subject upon completion of the study to assess motivation, knowledge of the direction in which blood pressure changes were being reinforced, and what cognitive processes were used to effect changes.

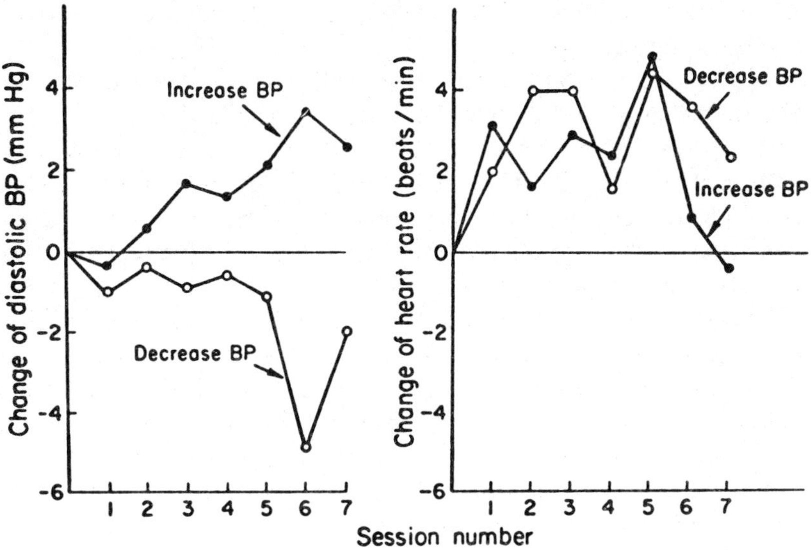

Figure 11-2 Average changes of diastolic pressure (left) and heart rate (right) for the increase and decrease groups. From Pickering, T. G., Brucker, B., Dworkin, B. R. and Miller, N. E.: Learned voluntary control of diastolic pressure in severely paralyzed patients. Manuscript submitted for publication. Reproduced with the permission of the senior author.

Figure 11-2 illustrates the mean changes in diastolic blood pressure and heart rate, as a result of training, for the six subjects who completed all seven sessions.

Separation between the groups (those subjects trying to increase their blood pressure and those attempting to decrease it) became increasingly marked for blood pressure but not for heart rate. By the fifth session it was apparent that some of the subjects were learning to change their blood pressure during the first thirty seconds of each trial. During Sessions six and seven, the first thirty seconds of a trial was used as a baseline period during which the subject rested and the tone was off. In the majority of cases, the pressure continued to change throughout the two-minute trial. Learned differences of diastolic pressure between the two groups was significant during both of these sessions. The increase group showed changes of 3.5 mm/Hg, and the decrease group had changes of -5.0 mm/Hg and -2.0 mm/Hg respectively for these two sessions.

Heart rate increased during the trials for both the increase and the decrease group, particularly during the early stages. There were no significant increases between the two groups at any stage, although significant increases were noted during the second and the fifth sessions for both groups combined.

There was no significant tendency for blood pressure to change during baseline periods when the subjects were not trying to change it. There were no consistent differences between baseline pressures at the beginning and end of each session, indicating that there was not a tendency for learned changes in blood pressure to carry over from one trial to the next during the course of an experimental session.

Subsequent experiments were conducted to try and determine the mechanisms used by the subjects in attempting to change their blood pressure. The effects of muscle tension were examined, and it was learned that for the increase group, while the subjects did not have the strength to contract their muscles, attempted contraction alone produced a marked rise in diastolic pressure and heart rate in one subject. The subjects in the decrease group were less likely to change their blood pressure through skeletal muscle contractions. While they could have tensed their muscles during the initial thirty seconds of each trial and then relaxed during the remainder of the trial, thereby giving the impression of decreased blood pressure, the pretrial baseline pressures were not any higher than the pressures for the baseline periods at the beginning and the end of each trial. Skeletal responses, therefore, do not appear responsible for the subjects' autonomic learning in this study.

When the possibility that respiratory responses may have been responsible for the changes in diastolic pressure was investigated it was found not to be the case. All three of the subjects who learned to change their diastolic blood pressure significantly were able to reproduce their learned changes without any change of

pCO_2. Thus, respiratory activity was not responsible for the learned behavior.

Only two of the subjects correctly identified the direction in which they were trying to change their blood pressure, and only one of these was able to do so, i.e. increase pressure. This subject used visual imagery to produce the changes. The other subjects had concentrated on the tone, or had relaxed.

The results obtained by Pickering et al. demonstrate that, through biofeedback procedures, small but reliable changes of diastolic blood pressure can be achieved by persons with nearly total neuromuscular paralysis.

This series of experiments raises several important questions, one of the most interesting of which is: How did the subjects do what they did, i.e. change their blood pressure? It was surprising to the investigators that attempting to contract atrophied muscles resulted in increases in blood pressure. Also notable is the fact that some of the subjects could increase their pressure without changing their heart rate. Hypoventilation, or holding the breath, can increase diastolic pressure, but none of the subjects did this, and one even exhibited a tendency towards hyperventilation. While muscle relaxation can result in decreased blood pressure, all of the subjects had severe muscular paralysis and atrophy, making this an unlikely explanation for the results.

As a conclusion, it appears, that each subject will use whatever mechanism he can in order to produce the desired response, and that this varies from person to person in different circumstances. There seems to be no definitive answer, as yet, as to how a paralyzed individual produces changes in his blood pressure.

* * * * *

Brucker and Ince (1975) employed biofeedback therapeutically to treat postural hypotension in a patient with a spinal cord injury. The subject was a thirty-one-year-old male with a complete lesion at the T_3 level of the spinal cord, secondary to a gunshot wound which occurred three years prior to his participation in the study.

He had been on an active rehabilitation program, including

intensive physical therapy, primarily for strengthening of his shoulder muscles and upper extremities. After considerable effort, the patient was fitted with long leg braces preparatory to crutch walking. However, each time he stood up, an exaggerated hypotension caused him to become dizzy, and frequently, to faint. Despite persistent efforts by the patient and his physical therapists, he was unable to remain in an upright position without vertigo and syncope occurring. His physical therapists contacted the psychologists concerning the problem, and it was decided to attempt to train him, through biofeedback, to learn to increase his blood pressure. At this time, diastolic readings, taken during the patient's attempts to stand, were below 30 mm/Hg.

A standard clinical sphygmomanometer and a standard clinical stethoscope, placed on the brachial artery, were used to measure both systolic and diastolic pressures. All measures were obtained clinically, i.e. by inflating the cuff above the systolic pressure level and then slowly deflating it while listening for the Korotkoff sound. Feedback of blood pressure levels was given to the patient verbally, by the experimenters who informed him of the readings.

The patient was seen for twelve 1-hour sessions, four days per week. Each session consisted of two 5-minute trials during which he tried to raise the level of his blood pressure. A three-minute rest period followed each trial. Measures of systolic and diastolic blood pressure were taken every sixty seconds, and these were reported to the patient. The patient was informed when a trial was about to begin, and that the experimenter would tell him when to start trying to increase his blood pressure. Then the readings were taken, the patient was told what they were, and he was instructed to try and raise his pressure. In addition to informing him of the readings every sixty seconds, the experimenter gave him information regarding the direction and magnitude of change in blood pressure since the previous reading, and told him the reading at the beginning of each trial. Verbal praise and encouragement also were given to the patient for increases in blood pressure.

At the end of each trial, the patient was told to stop trying to raise his blood pressure. During the rest period, systolic and diastolic measures were obtained every sixty seconds. While the patient rested, the magnitude and direction of the blood pressure changes which had occurred during the previous trial were discussed with him, and he was asked whether or not he was able to detect any changes which had taken place and, if so, by what means.

Prior to the initiation of experimental procedures, when the nature and purpose of the study had been explained to the patient, he had been told that he was to try and increase his blood pressure, on command, by concentrating on increased pressure without tensing his muscles or altering his respiration in any way.

Changes in blood pressure which occurred during the experimental trials were determined by comparing the last measure

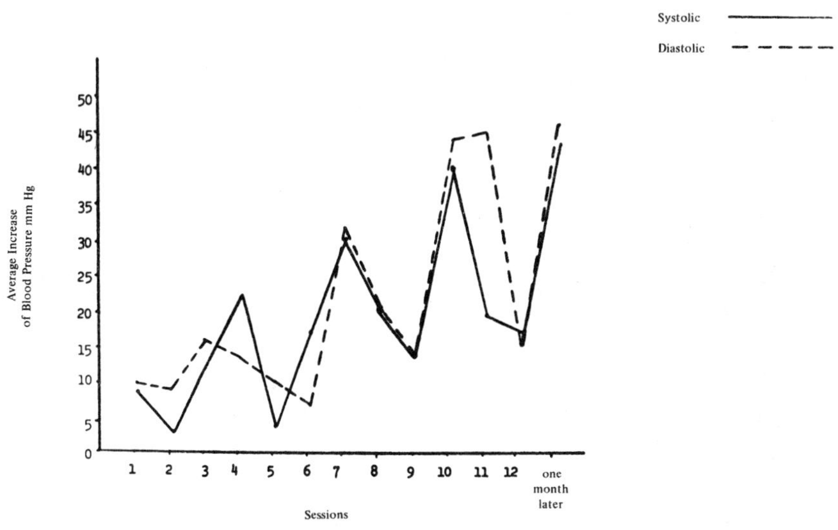

Figure 11-3 Mean increases in blood pressure during conditioning sessions. From Brucker, B. S. and Ince, L. P.: The application of biofeedback as a treatment for postural hypotension in a spinal cord lesion patient. Paper presented at the Annual Session of the American Congress of Rehabilitation Medicine, Atlanta, 1975.

Reproduced with the permission of the senior author and the American Congress of Rehabilitation Medicine.

obtained at the end of a trial with the measure which immediately preceded the instruction to the patient to increase his pressure for that trial. The change of blood pressure was calculated in this manner for both systolic and diastolic pressures.

Figure 11-3 shows the mean increases in both systolic and diastolic blood pressure for each of the twelve training sessions and for an additional session which was conducted one month following termination of the study. While considerable variation in the magnitude of the changes is apparent, the changes were consistently in the direction of increased blood pressure, and the mean magnitude of these changes increased with training. During the first and second sessions, the patient could attain changes of only up to 10 mm/Hg, but during the eleventh session he was able to achieve increases as great as 48 mm/Hg. An additional session,

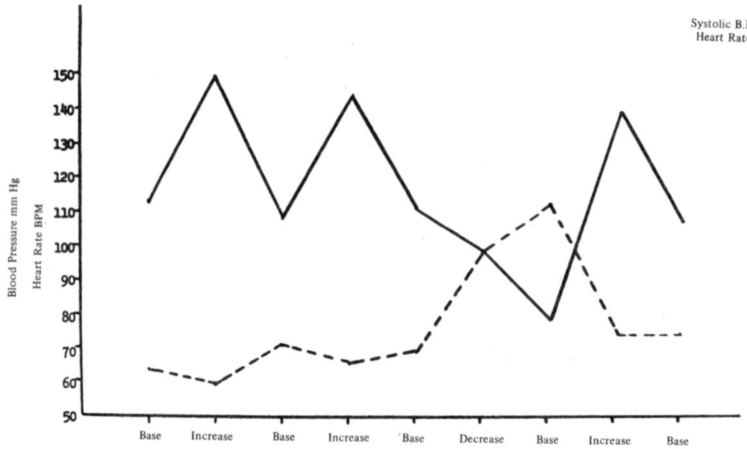

Figure 11-4 Systolic blood pressure and heart rate after conditioning. From Brucker, B. S. and Ince, L. P.: The application of biofeedback as a treatment for postural hypotension in a spinal cord lesion patient. Paper presented at the Annual Session of the American Congress of Rehabilitation Medicine, Atlanta, 1975.

Reproduced with the permission of the senior author and the American Congress of Rehabilitation Medicine.

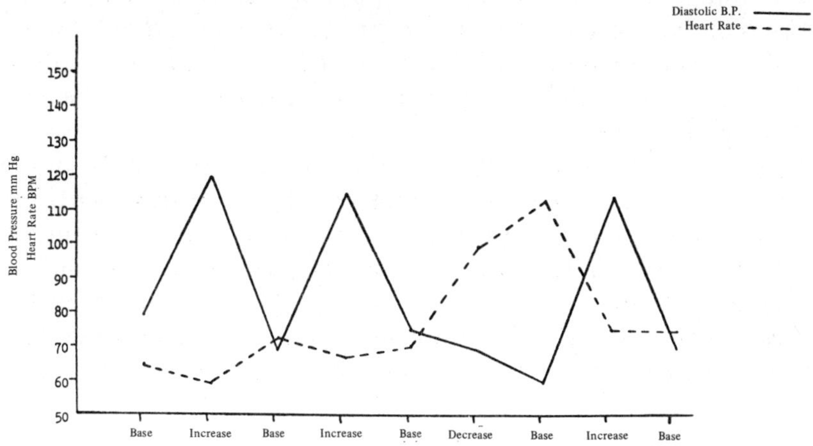

Figure 11-5 Diastolic blood pressure and heart rate after conditioning. From Brucker, B. S. and Ince, L. P.: The application of biofeedback as a treatment for postural hypotension in a spinal cord lesion patient. Paper presented at the Annual Session of the American Congress of Rehabilitation Medicine, Atlanta, 1975.

Reproduced with the permission of the senior author and the American Congress of Rehabilitation Medicine.

conducted one month post-training, revealed that the patient still was able to raise his blood pressure as much as 48 mm/Hg although no training had been conducted during this interim period and the patient had practiced his newly learned ability on his own.

During the experimental sessions, the patient developed certain sensations of high and low blood pressure, which he "felt" in his head. Feelings of dizziness signalled low blood pressure, and a feeling of pressure and a pulse beat in his head, accompanied by sweating, indicated high blood pressure. The patient utilized these sensations as feedback for his efforts to increase his pressure during the month's hiatus.

Figures 11-4 and 11-5 present the systolic and diastolic blood pressures, respectively, as well as the associated heart rate for trials during which the patient tried to increase and decrease his blood pressure, and for the rest intervals during the additional session.

The data reveals how reliably the patient was able to change his blood pressure on command. It is interesting to note that his heart rate consistently decreased during the trials when he was voluntarily increasing his blood pressure, and increased when he lowered his pressure.

Figures 11-6 and 11-7 illustrate the systolic and diastolic blood pressure measures obtained before and after training, with the patient trying to increase his pressure in a sitting and then a standing position. It is apparent that the patient's learned ability to raise his blood pressure had a dramatic effect on sustaining his pressure at a desirable level during conditions which otherwise would produce exaggerated hypotension. Prior to training with

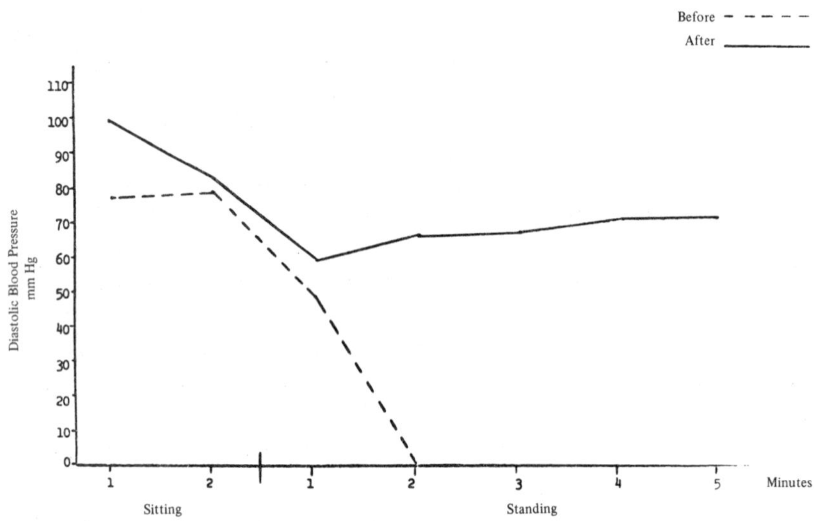

Figure 11-6 Average systolic blood pressure while standing after conditioning. From Brucker, B. S. and Ince, L. P.: The application of biofeedback as a treatment for postural hypotension in a spinal cord lesion patient. Paper presented at the Annual Session of the American Congress of Rehabilitation Medicine, Atlanta, 1975.

Reproduced with the permission of the senior author and the American Congress of Rehabilitation Medicine.

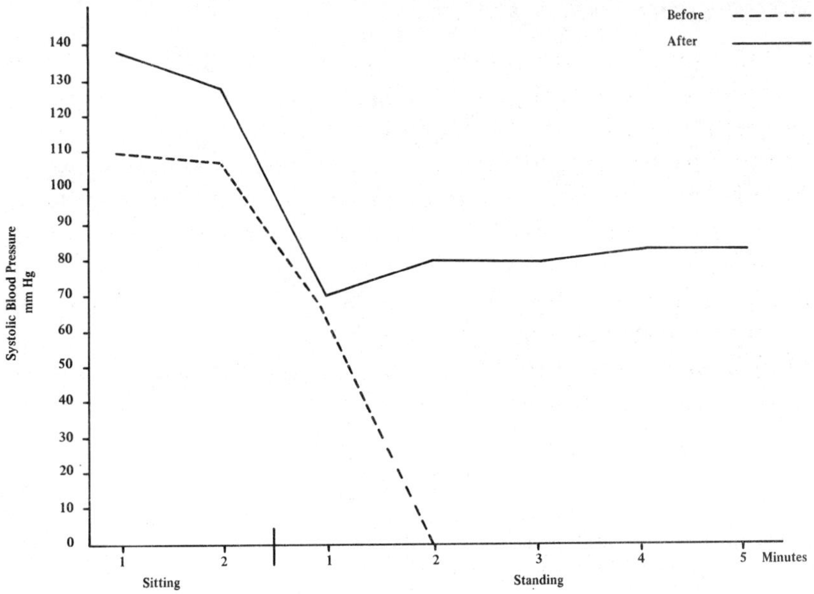

Figure 11-7 Average diastolic blood pressure while standing after conditioning. From Brucker, B. S. and Ince, L. P.: The application of biofeedback as a treatment for postural hypotension in a spinal cord lesion patient. Paper presented at the Annual Session of the American Congress of Rehabilitation Medicine, Atlanta, 1975.

Reproduced with the permission of the senior author and the American Congress of Rehabilitation Medicine.

biofeedback, standing for as brief a period of time as two minutes caused decreases in both systolic and diastolic pressure to the point of syncope. After conditioning, the patient was able to overcome this effect.

Subsequent attempts at standing, without the patient voluntarily increasing his blood pressure, resulted in an identical lowering of pressure as did the pretraining attempts. This suggests that the sustained blood pressure level after the experimental period was due to volitional control and not to overall adjustment.

With increased passage of time, the patient only had to concentrate on raising his blood pressure periodically as he ambulated with crutches. Eventually, he became able to ambulate and/or remain standing without the need to consciously raise his blood pressure at periodic intervals.

The investigations reported in this chapter, while raising many questions, illustrate that biofeedback can be utilized in therapeutic ways, even when dealing with severe disabilities. As mentioned at the outset of this section, biofeedback must still be viewed as largely experimental, yet many clinicians and researchers are demonstrating reliably that it holds much promise for treating a number of the problems of rehabilitation patients. As procedures are refined and more knowledge is gained, particularly concerning the mechanisms through which learning occurs with biofeedback, the future is likely to see increasing incorporation of these techniques into rehabilitative therapy programs.

REFERENCES

Blanchard, E. B. and Young, L. D.: Clinical applications of biofeedback training. *Arch Gen Psychiatry, 30*:573, 1974.

Brucker, B. S. and Ince, L. P.: The application of biofeedback as a treatment for postural hypotension in a spinal cord lesion patient. Paper presented at the Annual Session of the American Congress of Rehabilitation Medicine, Atlanta, 1975.

Brudny, J., Grynbaum, B. B. and Korein, J.: Spasmodic torticollis: Treatment by feedback display of the EMG. *Arch Phys Med Rehabil, 55*:403, 1974.

Brudny, J., Korein, J., Friedmann, L. W., Grynbaum, B. B., Weinstein, S. and Frankel, G.: Therapeutic applications of electromyography in the practice of rehabilitation medicine. Paper presented at the Annual Meeting of the American Congress of Rehabilitation Medicine, San Francisco, 1974.

Cleeland, C. S.: Behavioral technics in the modification of spasmodic torticollis. *Neurology, 23*:1241, 1973.

Craik, R. Wannstedt, Gunilla and Hesson, L.: Biofeedback and therapy. Paper presented at symposium entitled Lower Extremity and Spinal Orthotics as Related to Patient Evaluation and Therapeutic Training, Philadelphia, 1974.

Di Cara, L. V., Barber, T. X., Kamiya, J., Miller, N. E., Shapiro, D. and Stoyva, J. (Eds.) *Biofeedback and Self-Control.* Chicago, Aldine, 1974.

Di Cara, L. V. and Miller, N. E.: Heart-rate learning in the noncurarized state, transfer to the curarized state and subsequent retraining in the noncurarized state. *Amer J Physiol, 4*:621, 1969.

Herman, R.: Augmented sensory feedback in the control of limb movement. Paper presented at the Third Annual Meeting of the Society for Neuroscience, San Diego, 1973. In neural organization and its relevance to prosthetics. Miami, Symposia Specialists, 1973.

Herman, R.: Biofeedback. Paper presented at the Regional Training Session on Cerebral Palsy, Harrisburg, 1974a.

Herman, R.: Application of biofeedback to rehabilitation medicine. Paper presented at the Post-Graduate Program on Biofeedback Training in Physical Disabilities, Denver, 1974b.

Ince, L. P.: *The Rehabilitation Medicine Services*. Springfield, Thomas, 1974.

Jacobs, A. and Felton, G. S.: Visual feedback of myoelectric output to facilitate muscle relaxation in normal persons and patients with neck injuries. *Arch Phys Med Rehabil, 50*:34, 1969.

Pickering, T. G., Brucker, B. S., Dworkin, B. R. and Miller, N. E.: *Learned Voluntary Control of Diastolic Pressure in Severely Paralyzed Patients.* Manuscript submitted for publication.

Podivinsky, F.: Role of sensory and emotional inputs in mechanisms underlying involuntary motor activity. *Activ Nerv Sup Praha, 11*:19, 1969.

Taylor, D. R.: Electronic devices for the enhancement of rehabilitative therapy. Paper presented at Conference on Engineering Devices in Rehabilitation, Boston, 1974.

Wooldridge, C. P.: Biofeedback therapy for cerebral palsy children. Paper presented at Conference on Biofeedback Therapy in the Practice of Rehabilitation, Philadelphia, 1974.

Yates, A. J.: The application of learning theory to the treatment of tics. *J Abnorm Psychol, 56*:175, 1958.

SUPPLEMENTARY READING LIST

Amato, A., Hermsmeyer, C. A. and Kleinman, K. M.: Use of electromyographic feedback to increase inhibitory control of spastic muscles. *Phys Ther, 53*:1063, 1973.

Andrews, J. M.: Neuromuscular re-education of the hemiplegic with the aid of the electromyograph. *Arch Phys Med Rehabil, 45*:530, 1964.

Arsham, Diana S.: Applications of behavior modification techniques to the care of patients with pain and spasm from low back injuries. Paper presented at Conference on Medical Applications of Behavior Modification, San Francisco, 1975.

Barry, J. R.: Behavioral classification of the physically disabled. *Psychol Asp Disabil, 18*:136, 1971.

Basmajian, J. V., Kukulka, C. G., Narayan, M. G. and Takebe, K.: Biofeedback treatment of foot-drop after stroke compared with standard rehabilitation technique: Effects on voluntary control and strength. *Arch Phys Med Rehabil, 56*:231, 1975.

Berni, Rosemarian: Reinforcing behavior. *Am J Nurs, 71*:2180, 1971.

Berni, Rosemarian and Fordyce, W. E.: *Behavior Modification and the Nursing Process*. St. Louis, Mosby, 1973.

Biggs, S. And Bowman, J. T.: Applicability and efficacy of a behavioral approach to rehabilitation counseling. *J Appl Rehab Couns, 4*:239, 1973.

Birk, L. (Ed.): *Biofeedback: Behavioral Medicine*. New York, Grune and Stratton, 1973.

Birnbrauer, J. S.: Exploration of operant conditioning in physical therapy. Paper presented at the Annual Convention of the American Association on Mental Deficiency, Chicago, 1966.

Brookshire, R. H.: Speech pathology and the experimental analysis of behavior. *J Speech Hear Disord, 32*:215, 1967.

Brookshire, R. H.: Probability learning by aphasic subjects. *J Speech Hear Res, 12*:857, 1969.

Brookshire, R. H.: Control of "involuntary" crying behavior emitted by a multiple sclerosis patient. *J Communic Dis, 3*:171, 1970.

Brookshire, R. H.: Effects of delay of reinforcement on probability learning by aphasic subjects. *J Speech Hear Res, 14*:92, 1971.

Brookshire, R. H.: The use of consequences in speech pathology: Incentive and feedback functions. *J Communic Dis, 6*:88, 1973.

Brudny, J., Korein, J., Levidow, L., Grynbaum, B. B., Lieberman, A. and Friedmann, L. W.: Sensory feedback therapy as a modality of treatment in central nervous system disorders of voluntary movement. *Neurol, 24*:925, 1974.

Carney, Carolyn A.: Rehabilitation: a two-way street. The paraprofessional and behavior modification. Paper presented at the Annual Meeting of the Association for Advancement of Behavior Therapy, Miami Beach, 1970.

Cautela, J.: Behavior therapy and the aged. Paper presented at the Annual Meeting of the Eastern Psychological Association, Boston, 1967.

Cautela, J. R.: A classical conditioning approach to the development and modification of behavior in the aged. Paper presented at the Annual Convention of the American Psychological Association, San Francisco, 1968.

Chandler, L. S. and Adams, M. A.: Multiply handicapped child motivated for ambulation through behavior modification. *Phys Ther, 52*:399, 1972.

Connolly, K.: The application of operant conditioning to the measurement and development of motor skill in children. *Dev Med Child Neurol, 6*:679, 1968.

Croskey, Cheryl S. and Adams, M. R.: The experimental analysis of certain aspects of an aphasic's recovery. *J Communic Dis, 3*:177, 1970.

Cullen, J.: Behavior modification in cancer rehabilitation. Paper presented at Conference on Medical Applications of Behavior Modification, San Francisco, 1975.

Cushing, Martha: When counseling fails — then what? *J Rehabil, 35*:18, 1969.

Daly, D. A., Cantrell, R. P., Cantrell, M. L. and Aman, L. A.: Structuring speech therapy contingencies with an oral apraxic child. *J Speech Hear Disord, 37*:22, 1972.

Drash, P. W., Caldwell, Lynn R. and Leibowitz, J. M.: Correct and incorrect response rates as basic dependent variables in the operant conditioning of speech in non-verbal subjects. *Psychol Asp Disabil, 16*:17, 1970.

Duncan, P. K.: Modification of walking posture using basic principles of applied behavior analysis. *SALT: Sch Appl Learn Theory, 6*:1, 1974.

Engel, B. T.: Clinical applications of operant conditioning techniques in the control of cardiac arrhythmias. In Birk, L. (Ed.): *Biofeedback: Behavioral Medicine*. New York, Grune and Stratton, 1973.

Evans, R. I.: Social psychology of communication: a crucial factor in applying behavior modification principles to cancer rehabilitation. Paper presented at Conference on Medical Applications of Behavior Modification, San Francisco, 1975.

Feldman, M. C. and Di Scipio, W. J.: Integrating physical therapy with behavior therapy. A case study. *Phys Ther, 52*:1283, 1972.

Filby, Yasuko and Edwards, A. E.: An application of automated teaching methods to test and teach form discrimination to aphasics. *J Prog Instr, 2*:25, 1963.

Fitch, J. L.: Treatment of a case of cerebral palsy with hearing impairment. *J Speech Hear Disord, 37*:373, 1972.

Fordyce, W. E.: Automated training system for wheelchair pushups. *Public*

Health Rpts, 83:527, 1968.

Fordyce, W. E.: Operant conditioning as a treatment method in management of selected chronic pain problems. *Northwest Med, 8*:580, 1970.

Fordyce, W. E.: Behavioral methods in rehabilitation. In Neff, W. S. (Ed.): *Rehabilitation Psychology*. Washington, APA, 1971.

Fordyce, W. E.: An operant conditioning method for managing chronic pain. *Postgrad Med, 53*:123, 1973.

Fordyce, W. E.: Rehabilitation and behavioral science. Paper presented at the Annual Convention of the American Psychological Association, New Orleans, 1974.

Foss, B. M.: Operant conditioning in the control of movements. *Dev Med Child Neurol, 8*:331, 1966.

Friedlander, B. Z.: Automated techniques employing audio/visual reinforcement in perceptual evaluation and behavior development with retarded and disabled infants and children. Paper presented at the Fourth International Seminar on Special Education, Cork, Ireland, 1969.

Friedlander, B. Z.: Automated evaluation of selective listening in language-impaired and normal infants and young children. *Matern Child Health Exch, 1*:9, 1971.

Friedlander, B. Z., Kamin, Phyllis and Hesse, G. W.: Operant therapy for prehension disabilities in moderately and severely retarded young children. *Train Sch Bull, 71*:101, 1974.

Goodkin, R.: Improving verbal and motor behavior in hemiplegics through operant conditioning. Paper presented at the Annual Convention of the American Psychological Association, New York, 1966.

Gray, E. R.: Conscious control of motor units in a tonic muscle. *Am J Phys Med, 50*:34, 1971.

Halberstam, J. L. and Zaretsky, H. H.: Learning capacities of the elderly and brain-damaged. *Arch Phys Med Rehabil, 50*:133, 1969.

Hall, R. G.: Behavior modification and geriatrics: values, goals and ethics. Paper presented at the Annual Meeting of the Association for Advancement of Behavior Therapy, Miami Beach, 1973.

Halpern, H.: Effect of stimulus variables on dysphasic verbal errors. *Percept Mot Skills, 21*:291, 1965.

Hartley, R. B.: Pain and medication: a behavioral approach. Paper presented at Conference on Medical Applications of Behavior Modification, San Francisco, 1975.

Hartley, R. B.: Application of behavior modification techniques to the care of stroke patients. Paper presented at Conference on Medical Applications of Behavior Modification, San Francisco, 1975.

Haughton, E.: Shaping participation in occupational therapy. Paper presented at the Third International Congress World Federation of Occupational Therapists, Boston, 1962.

Holbrook, A., Rolnick, M. I. and Bailey, C. W.: Treatment of vocal abuse disorders using a vocal intensity controller. *J Speech Hear Disord, 39*:298,

1974.

Holland, Audrey: Some applications of behavioral principles to clinical speech problems. *J Speech Hear Disord, 32*:11, 1967.

Holland, Audrey: The use of programmed instruction with aphasics. Paper presented at the Annual Meeting of the American Congress of Rehabilitation Medicine, Chicago, 1968.

Holland, Audrey I. and Matthews, J.: Application of teaching machine concepts to speech pathology and audiology. *J Am Sp Hear Assoc, 5*:474, 1963.

Ince, L. P.: Applications of experimental psychology in a chronic disease setting: behavior modification. Paper presented at Fourth Annual Course on Remedial Techniques for Cognitive and Perceptual Difficulties in Brain Damaged Persons, New York, 1974.

Ince, L. P.: Biofeedback in rehabilitation. Paper presented at Conference on Medical Applications of Behavior Modification, San Francisco, 1975.

Ince, L. P.: Applications of behavior modification techniques to the care of patients with spinal cord injuries. Paper presented at Conference on Medical Applications of Behavior Modification, San Francisco, 1975.

Johnson, H. E.: Biofeedback and its application to rehabilitation. Paper presented at the Annual Assembly of the Academy of Physical Medicine and Rehabilitation, San Francisco, 1974.

Johnson, H. E. and Garton, W. H.: Muscle re-education in hemiplegia by use of electromyographic device. *Arch Phys Med Rehabil, 54*:320, 1973.

Kolderie, M. L.: Behavior modification in the treatment of children with cerebral palsy. *Phys Ther, 51*:1083, 1971.

Korein, J., Levidow, L. and Brudny, J.: Self-regulation of EEG and EMG activity using biofeedback as a therapeutic tool. *Electroencephalogr Clin Neurophysiol, 36*:222, 1974.

Kutner, J.: Discrimination conditioning and severe head injury. Paper presented at the Annual Convention of the American Psychological Association, New Orleans, 1974.

Lahey, B. (Ed.): *The Modification of Languuge Behavior.* Springfield, Thomas, 1972.

Lane, H. L. and Moore, D. J.: Reconditioning a consonant discrimination in aphasics: An experimental case history. *J Speech Hear Disord, 27*:232, 1962.

Larsen, L. A.: Behavior modification with the multihandicapped. *New Outlook Blind, 64*:6, 1970.

Leslie, G. (Ed.): *Behavior Modification in Rehabilitation Facilities.* Hot Springs, Arkansas Rehabilitation and Research Center, 1968.

Lindsley, O. R.: Geriatric behavioral prosthetics. In Kastenbaum, R. (Ed.): *New Thoughts On Old Age.* New York, Springer, 1964.

MacDonald, Marian L. and Butler, Audry K.: Reversal of helplessness: Producing walking behavior in nursing home wheelchair residents using behavior modification procedures. *J Gerontol, 29*:97, 1974.

Madison, H. L. and Herring, Marjorie: An experimental study of motivation.

Am J Occup Ther, 14:253, 1960.

Maher, K. R.: Auditory feedback of muscle action potentials: Applications to spasticity and athetosis. In *Productivity and the Cerebral Palsied.* Sydney, Australia, Centre Industries, 1972.

Marinacci, A. A. and Horande, M.: Electromyogram in neuromuscular re-education. *Bull Los Angeles Neurol Soc, 25*:57, 1960.

Marshall, R. C.: The effects of response-contingent punishment upon a defective articulation response. *J Speech Hear Disord, 35*:236, 1970.

Martin, J. E. and Sachs, D. A.: The effects of visual feedback on the fine motor behavior of a deaf cerebral palsied child. *J Nerv Ment Dis, 157*:59, 1973.

McDaniel, J. W.: *Physical Disability and Human Behavior.* New York, Pergamon, 1969.

McReynolds, Leija V.: Operant conditioning for investigating speech sound discrimination in aphasic children. *J Speech Hear Res, 9*:519, 1969.

McReynolds, Leija V.: Contingencies and consequences in speech therapy. *J Speech Hear Disord, 35*:12, 1970.

Meyerson, L., Michael, J. L., Mowrer, O. H., Osgood, C. E. and Staats, A. W.: Learning, behavior and rehabilitation. In Lofquist, L. H. (Ed.): *Psychological Research and Rehabilitation.* Washington, APA, 1960.

Michael, J.: Behavioral approaches to rehabilitation. Paper presented at Stanford University Medical School, 1963.

Michael, J. L.: Rehabilitation. In Neuringer, C. and Michael, J. L. (Eds): *Behavior Modification in Clinical Psychology.* New York, Appleton-Century-Crofts, 1970.

Miller, R. H. and Keith, R. A.: Behavioral mapping in a rehabilitation hospital. *Rehab Psychol, 20*:148, 1973.

Mowrer, D. E.: The management of consequent events in speech therapy. *Educ Technol, April*:58, 1971.

Mulholland, T.: Feedback electroencephalography. *Activas Nervosa Superior, 10*:410, 1968.

Nergardh, A., von Hedenberg, C., Hellstrom, B. and Ericsson, N.: Continence training of children with neurogenic bladder dysfunction. *Dev Med Child Neurol, 16*:47, 1974.

Osborne, J. G. and Wageman, R. M.: Some operant conditioning techniques and their use in schools for the deaf. *Am Ann Deaf, 114*:741, 1969.

Patterson, C. H.: Behavior modification in rehabilitation: A consideration of its values and limitations. *Rehab Res Pract Rev, 2*:1, 1970.

Pigott, R. A.: Behavior modification and control in rehabilitation. *J Rehabil, 35*:12, 1969.

Pineda, M., Barlow, H. and Turner, B. B.: Treatment of a severe speech disorder by behavior modification: A case study. *J Behav Ther Exp Psychiat, 2*:203, 1971.

Potvin, A. R., Tourtellotte, W. W., Pew, R. W., Albers, J. W., Henderson, W. G. and Snyder, Dorothy N.: Motivation and learning in the quantitative examination of neurological function. *Arch Phys Med Rehabil., 54*:432,

1973.

Roll, J. L.: Manipulation of fundamental frequency in functional voice disorders by application of reinforcement principles. Unpublished Doctoral Dissertation, Florida State University, 1969.

Rugal, R. S., Mattingly, J., Eichinger, M. and May, J.: The use of operant conditioning with physically disabled children. *Am J Occup Ther, 25*:247, 1971.

Sailor, W., Guess, D. and Baer, D. M.: Functional language for verbally deficient children. *Ment Retard, June*:27, 1973.

Salzinger, K.: Behavior theory and problems of the deaf. *Am Ann Deaf, 115*:459, 1970.

Salzinger, K., Feldman, R. S., Cowan, Judith E. and Salzinger, Suzanne: Operant conditioning of verbal behavior in two young speech-deficient boys. In Krasner, L. and Ullmann, L. P. (Eds.): *Research in Behavior Modification: New Developments and Their Clinical Implications*. New York, Holt, Rinehart & Winston, 1965.

Schroeder, S. R. and Yarbrough C. C.: The principles of programmed instruction as a model for vocational rehabilitation. *J Appl Rehab Couns, 2*:180, 1972.

Shriberg, L. D.: A system for monitoring and conditioning modal fundamental frequency of speech. *J Appl Behav Anal, 4*:337, 1971.

Sidman, M., Stoddard, L. T., Mohr, J. P. and Leicester, J.: Behavioral studies of aphasia: Methods of investigation and analysis. *Neuropsychologia, 9*:119, 1971.

Silber, L. D. and Howard, Juanita: Systematic desensitization with a cerebral palsied college student. *Psychother: Theory, Res, Pract, 9*:17, 1972.

Simard, T. and Basmajian, J.: Methods in training the conscious control of motor units. *Arch Phys Med Rehabil, 48*:12, 1967.

Sloan, H. N. and MacAulay, Barbara D. (Eds): *Operant Procedures in Remedial Speech and Language Training*. New York, Houghton Mifflin, 1968.

Smith, K. E. and Hodgson, J.: The effects of systematic reinforcement on the speech discrimination responses of normal and hearing-impaired children. *J Audit Res, 10*:110, 1970.

Smith, K. U. and Henry, J. P.: Cybernetic foundations for rehabilitation. *Am J Phys Med, 46*:379, 1967.

Sterman, M. B.: Neurophysiologic and clinical studies of sensorimotor EEG biofeedback training: Some effects on epilepsy. *Semin Psychiat,* 5:507, 1973.

St. James-Roberts, I.: Why operant audiometry — A consideration of some shortcomings fundamental to the audiological testing of children. *J Speech Hear Disord, 37*:47, 1972.

Swann, D., van Wieringer, P. C. W. and Fokkema, S. D.: Auditory EMG feedback therapy to inhibit undesired motor activity. *Arch Phys Med Rehabil., 55*:251, 1974.

Walls, R.: Behavior modification and rehabilitation. *Rehab Couns Bull, 13*:173,

1969.

Walls, R. T.: A reinforcement contingency analysis of rehabilitation. *Rehab Res Pract Rev, 2*:29, 1971.

Weiner, A. E.: Speech therapy and behavior modification: a conspectus. *J Spec Educ, 3*:285, 1969.

Weiss, T. and Engel, B. T.: Operant conditioning of heart rate in patients with premature ventricular contractions. *Psychosom Med, 33*:301, 1971.

Wheeler, A. J. and Sulzer, Ruth: Operant training and generalization of a verbal response form in speech-deficient child. *J Appl Behav Anal, 3*:139, 1970.

Yoss, Kathe A. and Darley, F. L.: Therapy in developmental apraxia of speech. *Lang, Sp Hear Serv Sch, 5*:23, 1974.

Zifferblatt, S. M. and Dunbar, Jackie: Applying behavioral strategies to increase adherence with medical regimes. Paper presented at Conference on Medical Applications of Behavior Modification, San Francisco, 1975.

Zimmerman, J., Stuckey, T. E., Garlick, Betsy J. and Miller, Maurine: Effects of token reinforcement on productivity in multiply handicapped clients in a sheltered workshop. *Rehabil Lit, 30*:34, 1969.

AUTHOR INDEX